MIGRATION AND HEALTH

Migration and Health: Critical Perspectives offers a radical rethinking of the field by unsettling conventional ideas of mobility and borders to highlight the ways in which they produce health inequalities. Covering a wide range of topics, the text provides insight through a critical lens and proposes areas for intervention along with future research needs to address the health inequities that affect migrants. It illustrates how a critical perspective can deepen our understanding of the relationship between migration and health, which remains a defining global issue of our century.

The text employs a critical approach to examine the structural conditions of inequality and larger historical and political processes, recognizing that exclusionary bordering practices increasingly occur away from physical points of entry. It posits the concept of migration as complex, tangled, and multi-directional and underscores how migrant vulnerability can shape the lives of people in broader communities. Furthermore, it acknowledges diverse and intersectional standpoints, as well as shifting spatial and temporal influences. Chapters include coverage of health in transit; health care access and utilization; clinical encounters; communicable disease; labor and occupational health; gender and sexuality; immigration enforcement, detention, deportation; and the effects of forced displacement on refugee and asylum seeker health.

The text is useful for students and scholars of migration or health disparities seeking to understand how the two issues can be approached in a more holistic and critical way. It is further aimed at practitioners and policymakers who are interested in gaining familiarity with the structural conditions of inequality along with the larger historical and political processes that influence contemporary migration patterns.

Heide Castañeda is Professor of Anthropology at the University of South Florida. Her research areas include critical border studies, political and legal anthropology, medical anthropology, migration, migrant health, and citizenship, focusing on the U.S./Mexico border, Mexico, Germany, and Morocco.

CRITICAL APPROACHES TO HEALTH

The Routledge *Critical Approaches to Health* series aims to present critical, interdisciplinary books around psychological, social, and cultural issues related to health. Each volume in the series provides a critical approach to a particular issue or important topic, and is of interest and relevance to students and practitioners across the social sciences. The series is produced in association with the International Society of Critical Health Psychology (ISCHP).

Series Editors: Kerry Chamberlain & Antonia Lyons

Titles in the series:

Selling Immunity
Self, Culture and Economy in Healthcare and Medicine
Mark Davis

Embodied Trauma and Healing
Critical Conversations on the Concept of Health
Anna Westin

Migration and Health
Critical Perspectives
Heide Castañeda

For more information about this series, please visit: www.routledge.com/Critical-Approaches-to-Health/book-series/CRITHEA

MIGRATION AND HEALTH

Critical Perspectives

Heide Castañeda

Routledge
Taylor & Francis Group
LONDON AND NEW YORK

Cover image: © Getty Images

First published 2023
by Routledge
4 Park Square, Milton Park, Abingdon, Oxon OX14 4RN

and by Routledge
605 Third Avenue, New York, NY 10158

Routledge is an imprint of the Taylor & Francis Group, an informa business

British Library Cataloguing-in-Publication Data
A catalogue record for this book is available from the British Library

Library of Congress Cataloging-in-Publication Data
A catalog record has been requested for this book

ISBN: 978-1-138-49042-0 (hbk)
ISBN: 978-1-138-49043-7 (pbk)
ISBN: 978-1-003-30753-2 (ebk)

DOI: 10.4324/9781003307532

Typeset in Bembo
by Newgen Publishing UK

ⵓⵉⵏ ⵎⵓⵙⴹⴰⵀⴰ

CONTENTS

Series Editor Preface *xi*

1 Introduction 1
A Defining Global Issue 2
Critical Perspectives on Migrant Health 3
Empirical Challenges 5
Outline of the Book 7

2 Critical Perspectives on Migration and Health 12
Critical Border Studies 12
"Citizens" and "Migrants": Questions of Sovereignty, Il/Legality, and Inequality 14
Who Is a Migrant? Conceptual Pitfalls 17
Critical Perspectives on Health 21
"Healthy Migrant Effects" and Immigrant Health Paradoxes 25
Integration, Incorporation, and Acculturation 26
Pathogenic Conditions: From Behavioral Explanations to Structural Approaches 29
Conclusion 31

3 Health in Transit 32
Critical Approaches to Understanding Health in Transit 34
Violence of Border Controls and Production of Illegality 35
Forced Immobility and Stuckness 37
Smuggling and Trafficking 38

Respatialization of Border Controls: Externalization and Internalization Practices 39
Family Shifts and Separation through Migration 42
Cross-Border Ties: Implications for Health 43
Conclusion 45

4 Health Care Access and Utilization 46
Critical Approaches to Understanding Health Care Access and Utilization 48
Policy Frameworks Determining Access to Medical Care 49
Beyond Policy: Other Barriers to Access 52
Spillover Effects of Lack of Access 53
Health Providers as Gatekeepers, Street-Level Bureaucrats 54
Access via Charity Clinics, NGOs, and Nonprofits 55
Alternative Strategies for Treatment 56
Conclusion 57

5 The Clinical Encounter 58
Critical Approaches to Understanding the Clinical Encounter 60
Language and Communication Barriers 61
Patient-Centeredness, Diversity Sensitivity, and Cultural Competency 62
Structural Competency in the Clinic 64
Health "Literacy," Health Care Navigators, and Cultural Mediators 65
Diversity in the Clinical Workforce 66
"Migration Aware" Whole System Approaches 66
Conclusion 67

6 Communicable Disease 68
Critical Approaches to Understanding Communicable Disease 70
Legacies of Colonialism: The Diseased "Other," Border Controls, and Stigma 70
Tuberculosis: "Penalty" for the Ruthless Exploitation of Labor 72
HIV/AIDS: From Stigma to Specific Vulnerabilities for Migrants 73
COVID-19: Management of Human Mobility at the Global Scale 75
Conclusion 79

7 Labor and Occupational Health 80
Critical Approaches to Understanding Labor and Occupational Health 82
Occupational Hazards 85
Labor Abuses: Trafficking and Wage Theft 86

Worker Injury and Injustices 87
Demonstrating Deservingness and Legitimacy in the Medical Encounter 89
Conclusion 91

8 Gender, Sexuality, and Migrant Health 92
Critical Approaches to Understanding Gender, Sexuality, and Migrant Health 95
Shifts in Family Structures, Conjugal Relationships, and Gender Roles 95
Gender and Reproduction 96
Transnational Parenting 98
Migration and Masculinities 99
Sexual and Queer Migrations 99
Sexual Health 100
Intimate Partner Violence 101
Conclusion 101

9 Health Impacts of Enforcement, Detention, and Deportation 103
Critical Approaches to Understanding Health Impacts of Enforcement, Detention, and Deportation 105
Fear of Deportation and Effects on Mental and Emotional Health 107
Physical Health Impacts of Deportability 108
Effects on Health Service Access and Health-Seeking Behavior 108
Immigration Raids 109
Health Issues during the Detention or Deportation Process 109
Impacts of Deportation on Children 110
Impacts of Deportation on the Larger Family Unit 112
Impacts of Deportation on Communities 113
After Deportation: Return to Country of Origin 113
Conclusion 114

10 Forced Displacement: Refugee and Asylum Seeker Health 116
Critical Approaches to Understanding Forced Displacement: Refugee and Asylum Seeker Health 118
Protracted Displacement: Camps, Sustained Detention, and Reception Centers 119
Medical Examinations and "Proof" of Torture and Persecution 121
Health Care Access for Refugees and Asylum Seekers 121
Unique Health Needs of Refugees 123
Refugee Mental Health 124
Conclusion 125

11 Conclusion 127
Moving Forward with a Critical Agenda 127
The Search for Solutions 129
Future Research Imperatives 130

References *135*
Index *161*

SERIES EDITOR PREFACE

Critical Approaches to Health

Health is a major issue for people all around the world, and is fundamental to individual well-being, personal achievements, and satisfaction, as well as to families, communities, and societies. It is also embedded in social notions of participation and citizenship. Much has been written about health, from a variety of perspectives and disciplines, but a lot of this writing takes a biomedical and causally positivist approach to health matters, neglecting the historical, social, and cultural contexts and environments within which health is experienced, understood, and practiced. It is timely for a new series of books that offer critical, social science perspectives on important health topics.

The *Critical Approaches to Health* series aims to provide new critical works by presenting interdisciplinary and theoretical writing about health, where matters of health are framed quite broadly. The series seeks to include books that range across important health matters, including general health-related issues (e.g., gender and media), major social issues for health (e.g., medicalization, obesity, and palliative care), particular health concerns (e.g., pain, doctor–patient interaction, health services, and health technologies), particular health problems (e.g., diabetes, autoimmune disease, and medically unexplained illness), or health for specific groups of people (e.g., the health of migrants, the homeless, and the aged), or combinations of these.

The series seeks above all to promote critical thought about health matters. By critical, we mean going beyond the critique of the topic and work in the field to more general considerations of power and benefit and, in particular, to addressing concerns about whose understandings and interests are upheld and whose are marginalized by the approaches, findings, and practices in these various domains of health. Such critical agendas involve reflections on what constitutes knowledge, how it is created, and how it is used. Accordingly, critical approaches consider epistemological and theoretical positioning, as well as issues of methodology and practice, and seek to examine how health is enmeshed within broader social relations and structures. Books within this series take up this challenge and seek to provide new insights and understandings by applying a critical agenda to their topics.

In this book, *Migration and Health: Critical Perspectives,* Heide Castañeda delivers a challenging account of migration, in its diverse forms, and the variety of ways in which it relates to and impacts on health. The book offers a wide-ranging, multidisciplinary account of migration and health, synthesizing scholarship on a range of aspects of migration that are not usually considered together. She explicitly focuses on the social origins of illness, and how inequality, poverty, institutional constraints, and violence contribute to health disparities. Through her critical approach, Castañeda rethinks standard ideas about migration, mobility, and borders and problematizes taken-for-granted understandings. She focuses on the framing of, and assumptions made about, the origins and reasons for migration, as well as the huge social and policy implications of these framings. She then explores what happens to migrants in their new country; the processes of institutional, economic, and political marginalization that occur; and the consequences for their health and well-being.

Specific chapters address the theorization of key issues, migration, borders, citizenship, and sovereignty; the effects of transit and borders on migrants' health; how policies create deservingness, discrimination, and obligation, limiting access to health care; how health care systems fail to meet the needs of migrants; how migrants are linked to communicable diseases and how this limits health care treatment; how migrants are disadvantaged in terms of work, laboring in 3D (dirty, demanding, and dangerous) jobs and the implication of this work for health; how migrant health is shaped by gender and sexuality, with implications for reproduction, parenting, and citizenship; the impacts of immigration enforcement, detention, and deportation on the health of migrants, their families, and their communities; and the complexities that surround refugees and asylum seekers in obtaining legitimacy and accessing health care. The chapters are illustrated with effective case studies that illustrate and inform the arguments offered.

Throughout the book, Heide Castañeda consistently provides perspectives on migration and health that go beyond individual concerns to consider the broader social, political, and economic structural factors that drive issues of citizenship, inequality, poverty, entitlement, deservingness, stigma, discrimination, and access to care. This perspective allows Castañeda to offer a radical rethinking of migration and health, critically assessing conventional understandings of migration processes. She considers how policies, regulations, laws, institutional structures, and administrative systems were developed – and function best – for some populations over others, and in ways that imperil migrants, and impact and shape their health care and health outcomes. In short, this book challenges conventional ideas of migration, mobility, and borders: it rejects binary oppositions, such as citizens/

foreigners, natives/migrants, insiders/outsiders, illness/wellness; it rethinks notions of spatialities and temporalities around migration; and it embeds scholarship within complex histories of inequalities. The book provides an outstanding, original addition to the *Critical Approaches to Health* series on a topic with strong contemporary salience.

Kerry Chamberlain and Antonia Lyons
February 2022

1

INTRODUCTION

Far back enough in time, we are all migrants. Migration is part of what it is to be human, with population movements shaping the globe throughout the history of our species as a fundamental impulse to seek out better living conditions, whether that means safety and security, adequate resources, or a healthier environment. The experience of migration affects every aspect of daily life, requiring a complete realignment that can result in substantial social, economic, and health consequences. While recognized as a global health priority, the relationship between migration and health remains poorly understood because it is deeply entangled with other social and political conditions and experiences of marginality. Thus, to understand migrant health, we must first understand large-scale forces, including global inequality, political instability, economic insecurity, and climate change.

Migration and Health: Critical Perspectives calls for a radical rethinking by unsettling ideas about migration, mobility, and borders to explore the ways in which they produce health inequalities. It asks the reader to critically assess conventional wisdom and discourse about migration processes, as well as reconsider the ways in which health care and other institutional structures marginalize some populations in relation to others. A critical approach is attentive to structural conditions of inequality and larger historical and political processes; recognizes that many exclusionary bordering practices occur away from physical points of entry; conceptualizes migration as complex, tangled, and multidirectional; understands that migrant vulnerability shapes the lives of people in wider communities; and acknowledges diverse and intersectional standpoints, as well as shifting spatial and temporal influences. This book provides insights from a critical perspective, covering a wide breadth of topics as well as proposed areas of intervention and an analysis of future research needs to tackle the health inequities that affect migrants globally.

DOI: 10.4324/9781003307532-1

A Defining Global Issue

Migration has become a defining global issue of our century, even though the proportion of the world's migrants has remained relatively consistent over the past three decades at around 3.6% (International Organization for Migration [IOM] 2022). However, the scale and pace of mobility has been accelerated by technology and globalization processes, while economic inequalities, political conflicts, natural disasters, and environmental change have caused more people to leave their homelands. As a result, migrations are now much more frequent, more rapid, and to more distant places. We are currently witnessing the highest ever-recorded number of international migrants at 281 million, a swift increase from 173 million at the turn of the century (IOM 2022). If we include internal displacement, the number rises to more than one billion migrants worldwide, or one in seven people. And of course, the impacts reach beyond this figure to include millions more, as families and wider social networks are separated by borders, and labor markets become increasingly entangled within the wider global political economy (Thomas 2016).

While migration is a usual, frequent, and patterned part of the human experience, it is far from "natural." To gloss over the root causes of population movements would be an injustice to the people affected by them. Some of the highest levels of forced displacement on record are occurring today, with 84 million people leaving their homes worldwide, including approximately 26.6 million refugees and 4.4 million asylum seekers (UNHCR 2021). Globally, people continue to be displaced by various combinations of violence, choice, and circumstance, challenging the conventional relationship between "voluntary" migrants, who choose to cross borders in search of opportunity, and "involuntary" migrants, who are forced to flee in search of physical security. "Voluntary" movements themselves are almost always the result of economically violent circumstances that have obstructed life chances; thus, rather than easily characterized through this binary, the causes of migration must be thought of as complex and located along a spectrum (Yarris & Castañeda 2015).

In addition to the mobility of populations, *immobility* has become an important feature of contemporary migration. The COVID-19 pandemic fundamentally shifted the management of human mobility and became another "great disrupter" of migration worldwide (IOM 2022). However, it is better understood as a continuation of prior bordering processes rather than as a unique event or complete transformation. For example, a major element of response involved drastic restrictions to freedom of movement despite the World Health Organization's (WHO) strong preference for borders to remain open. However, if we consider a broader understanding of "borders," as this book argues, we can more easily understand these current global processes, especially since much of the exclusionary bordering people experience today takes place away from physical points of entry. Nonetheless, the recent pandemic has shown us the degree to which health across the world is interconnected. As it unfolded, it highlighted contemporary forms of sociality, governance systems rooted in inequality, and the various scales of mobility and selective bordering processes that accompany them.

Critical Perspectives on Migrant Health

This book employs a critical perspective to understand migration as it relates to inequitable patterns of health and illness. A critical perspective is defined as one "explicitly considering the nature of knowledge generation, the paradigms in which it was generated, and the consequences of this in terms of what knowledge is produced, with whom, and who benefits from this knowledge" (Chamberlain & Lyons 2020: 431). This approach locates an "object" or topic of investigation – here, the health of migrants – within the historical, social, and cultural contexts in which now dominant assumptions have emerged. In doing so, it allows us to better understand how particular social and material conditions influence or constrain the issue (Chamberlain & Lyons 2021).

Critical perspectives ask us to radically rethink our understandings and how we arrived at them. Especially attentive to issues of social, political, and economic power, its exercise, and distribution, these approaches are uniquely able to examine which groups benefit and which are disadvantaged. By critically unsettling migrant health, we can question taken-for-granted views about migration and mobility, as well as health and illness, and productively interrogate concerns related to power, identity, disadvantage, and inequality. This book takes on the epistemic challenges of a critical approach by rejecting clean binary oppositions, such as those that emerge between citizens and foreigners, natives and migrants, insiders and outsiders, as well as binaries of ill health and wellness and disconnects between the social and biological. It also seeks to rethink spatialities and temporalities associated with migration – for example, by considering the importance of both interior and exterior sites of migration management, as well as disruptions of familiar temporal registers because of new political reconfigurations or states of emergency.

Critical perspectives encourage us to not simply decenter existing understandings and discourses but also broaden our lens by including multiple, diverse, and intersectional standpoints, including gender, race, ethnicity, sexuality, and other forms of marginalization. In doing so, we can better identify and push back against dominant ideologies and the ways in which meanings are produced. Following this kind of reflexive consideration, critical approaches also identify ways in which disparities may be eliminated to uplift the disadvantaged.

This book makes the case for a critical approach to migrant health, in particular how inequality, poverty, institutional constraints, and violence contribute to disparities in risk, access, treatment, and outcomes. It synthesizes current scholarship from this critical perspective, engaging with current interdisciplinary debates such as the relationship between macrolevel social determinants of health and individual-level agency; the impact of social and institutional contexts for well-being; the relative importance of social position; how national and local policies shape health disparities; and the significance of global discourses of human rights and humanitarianism. An explicitly critical framing focuses on the social origins of illness and the context that precedes them (Castañeda et al. 2015; Fleischman et al. 2015; Krieger 2013, 2016). Such an approach joins together aspects of migration studies that are not ordinarily studied together with health disparities, such as labor migration, detention, and social integration.

A critical perspective requires, first, a rethinking of ideas about migration and how we arrived at them. This book thus asks the reader to decenter and unsettle notions of migration, mobility, and borders to problematize conventional understandings and focus instead on the exercise and distribution of social, political, and economic power and how it produces inequality in the context of health. This process involves the exploration of alternative epistemologies and the need to broaden our lens to include multiple and intersectional standpoints. This is necessary to transform existing colonizing, hegemonic, and often racist assumptions about migration in order to genuinely reform health inequities (Dubal et al. 2021).

Second, we must understand the structural reasons behind people's displacement. How we frame the origins of migration has enormous social and policy implications. When migration is viewed as unusual, problematic, or even pathological, assumptions are carried over into policy and research practice. When migration is regarded as an expected and necessary response to various forms of violence, it can result in the development of equitable policies to address disparities. This response requires a recognition that the global patterns of inequality fostering migration are not based so much on cultural difference, but are instead rooted in broader colonial processes and their social, political, and economic conditions.

Third, we must recognize the institutional, economic, and political marginalization that continues after migrants arrive in a new country, based on complex histories of inequalities with even deeper historical and political roots. Global patterns of inequality continue to impact the experiences of migrants in receiving (or "host") countries. This book posits that the state's power to create forms of difference between citizens and migrants is the result of broader ongoing processes of globalization and colonialism. Patterns of morbidity and mortality follow inequities produced and reproduced by laws, policies, bureaucratic procedures, and institutions. Inequities in the well-being of migrants are heavily determined by exclusionary processes, discrimination and racism, isolation, and constructs of legal status. Social and institutional contexts shape individuals' lives in relation to employment in marginal and dangerous jobs, inadequate housing, food insecurity, and poor access to transportation and other resources, with consequences for overall well-being. These conditions frequently emerge from assumptions regarding the root causes of their migration, which shape ideas about how deserving of incorporation into a host society a particular migrant group should be.

In taking a critical perspective on the issue of migration and health, some of the major principles this book centers include the following:

- Looks for causes of ill health not in behavioral, cultural, or individual factors, but rather in structural conditions of inequality (and the larger historical and political processes that underlie those)

- Is explicitly attentive to social, political, and economic power, its exercise and distribution
- Acknowledges that migration is the result of broader globalization and colonialism processes that displace populations
- Includes multiple, diverse, and intersectional standpoints, as well as shifting spatial and temporal influences
- Recognizes that much of the exclusionary bordering people experience today takes place away from physical points of entry
- Rejects orderly binary oppositions in favor of alternative vocabularies that acknowledge complex, tangled, temporary, and intermediate experiences, situations, and spaces
- Recognizes that migration is not linear, unidirectional, or easily split into discrete "phases," as this implies stabile epistemic partitions between "here" and "there"
- Avoids studying migrants from the unproblematized standpoint of citizens, accounting for our own positionality and its role in intrinsic inequality
- Does not treat migration or mobility as abnormal, and sedentism as the norm
- Troubles "the border" as a natural or fixed object, acknowledging that borders transcend physical boundaries
- Recognizes human freedom of movement as fundamental instead of rendering migration as transgressive, exceptional, or pathological
- Does not uphold colonialist notions by implicitly positing the Global North as the only, primary, or preferred destination in migrant imaginations
- Is highly attentive to and explains terminology utilized and assures congruence with the variable of interest
- Avoids use of violent and militarized terms and dehumanizing language
- Recognizes that the health of migrants is significantly affected by inequality, poverty, institutional constraints, and violence in host countries, rather than an expression of conditions in countries of origin
- Understands that migrant vulnerability also shapes the health of non-migrants and communities connected to them
- Seeks ways to eliminate health disparities and uplift migrant populations

Empirical Challenges

One of the main arguments of this book is that migration is not linear, unidirectional, or easily broken into discrete phases. However, as a starting point, it is still useful to examine the various moments of the process and how they interact with issues of health, especially to understand methodological challenges (Wickramage et al. 2018). Across all these moments, race, ethnicity, gender, class, socioeconomic status, age, and biological predisposition additionally impact people's experiences of health and illness.

The health profile of, and epidemiologic situation in, the "home" community may play a relevant role in the "pre-migration" phase. The decision or necessity to migrate may be impacted by events that create trauma, including conflict, violence, torture, climate change, or economic depression. During the "movement" phase, health may be impacted negatively if the journey is arduous and dangerous, or as people make use of smugglers or face the anxiety and instability of overstaying a visa. Travel conditions themselves may be perilous and lack conditions for wellbeing (e.g., sanitation, nutrition). People may be vulnerable to violence, exploitation, and other abuses; they may travel alone, isolated and defenseless, or with a group, supporting one another. On the other hand, some migrants may travel in relative comfort, simply boarding an airplane and/or arriving with authorization to enter a host country, resulting in a wide variety of experiences.

Upon arrival, the role of national and local policies regarding both immigration and health is vital. Legal status often significantly affects access to services. "Othering" processes may exclude migrants and lead to exclusion, discrimination, marginalization, and exploitation. In addition, there may be conflicts with social values or language; the availability of services tailored to migrants varies widely. Finally, the separation from family members, friends, and other loved ones frequently has emotional and mental health impacts.

Of course, many migrants also return to their home countries (and very frequently more than once, sometimes seasonally, sometimes permanently). Wellbeing in these cases may be affected by the duration of absence, household factors such as debt, the character of ties to family and community, and the availability of services. Finally, the overall health profile of the "home" community may have changed significantly in the meantime as well and its impacts on wellbeing need to be accounted for.

Methodologically, the study of migration frequently involves striking an analytical balance between fluid and what may appear to be haphazard movement and the bounds of nationalist thought. There is a conceptual tendency in migration studies to naturalize the global regime of nation-states; it may be easy to forget that these are recent political constructions. This analytical bias, referred to as *methodological nationalism,* privileges the nation-state as the site for social processes, often to the neglect of other kinds of experiences. Studies that are posited from the epistemic perspective of the migrant-receiving country without explicit acknowledgement exemplify this bias (De Genova 2016). This is particularly problematic during times of heightened nativism and anti-immigrant racism. Alternatively, it is useful to consider that, in our current global system, there is no stabile epistemic partition between "here" and "there," and migrants are not simply dislocated, "displaced," or "uprooted" persons who demonstrate some form of "spatial disobedience" (De Genova 2016). This pitfall of located-ness leads to analyses of migrant health that emphasize simplistic abstractions about geographically determinate social and "cultural" difference.

The study of migrant health presents methodological challenges because migration is a dynamic and non-linear process. It can start and stop or take on circular patterns. As a result, it is not possible to rely on single measures of movement, as these metrics result in contradictory and non-comparable research findings (Vearey 2016). Another major issue is the causal identification of interconnections with specific health issues, complicated by mechanisms such as selection effects of who migrates in the first place, the role of socioeconomic and psychosocial factors, and how health impacts the experience of return. Complicating matters, surveillance systems rarely collect or disaggregate data according to migrant status. The definition of who is considered a migrant varies greatly and is often determined by national legislative, administrative, and policy factors. There is usually also a lack of data on specific migrant groups, such as those who are undocumented (Williams et al. 2016).

A major challenge associated with summarizing insights from multiple disciplines comes, of course, from their varied methodologies. Some studies of migrant health are analyses of national-representative surveys, or utilize a cross-sectional, randomized control case, or incidence/prevalence design. Others are primarily qualitative, including descriptive, ethnographic, and phenomenological approaches. Some employ mixed methods, using embedded or triangulation designs. Furthermore, given the diversity of study types, it is not surprising that sample sizes vary considerably across the existing literature. In general, available datasets contain great variability in denominators of citizenship, residency, and immigration status, making comparisons difficult. To account for immediate, long-term, and inter-generational impacts on health, research would ideally collect data during the different phases of migration (in the homeland, during transit, after migrating), but this is rarely possible. Instead, there is heavy reliance on retrospective measures and self-reporting. Methodological innovation is required, including, for instance, a life-course approach (Wickramage et al. 2018).

Bi- or multinational approaches to understanding migrant health can better offer critical insights into the processes affecting health outcomes, but these are rare (Handley & Sudhinaraset 2017). Some studies have collected primary data in border regions, but fewer have been conducted outside of these areas, which would add to understanding a broader range of migration experiences. While the availability of large datasets from multiple countries has increasingly allowed for comparisons, they are rarely able to provide much contextual information about the social and structural factors affecting health. They also do not allow for an in-depth look at the experiences of unique communities, such as Indigenous People, for whom we know that there are additional important factors affecting health. As noted earlier, there is also a widespread bias toward international rather than internal migration.

Outline of the Book

This book unfolds over eight topical chapters and a conclusion. Each chapter covers a major conceptual area and summarizes the extant literature. Since the combinations of multiple disciplines, variety of countries, and multiple critical lenses could easily result in disorganization, each chapter is structured in the following way: First, I offer a brief vignette based on my own research to introduce the topic. Next, I highlight major theoretical questions and conceptual debates, and explain what a critical perspective can add to major thematic areas.

This book covers a wide breadth of the topics, offering a foundation for anyone interested in current issues and debates within a variety of sociolegal contexts that produce their own forms of structural violence and opportunities for care. While it draws on examples from around the globe, the book focuses primarily on international migration to "developed" countries due to the large and robust literature that has emerged in what have historically been primary "host" countries. In recent decades, international migration has indeed become concentrated in a "shrinking pool of prime destination countries" (Czaika & Haas 2014: 283); nonetheless, existing scholarship is disproportionately focused on certain regions of the world. Thus, while internal migration (within a single country or region) and South-South migration (between low- and middle-income countries) have become increasingly important, there is less information about them included here. Nonetheless, it is important to note that in many parts of the world, internal migration far exceeds the number of cross-border migrants and can present even greater challenges for health systems and health equity (Vearey et al. 2017). Similarly, migration between countries of the "Global South" remain frequently invisible to researchers, policymakers, and the media, as attention is focused on migration to high-income countries (Wickramage et al. 2018). While acknowledged throughout, a full discussion of these omissions is regretful but necessary for the scope of the book's examination of displacement experiences and the specific influence of host-country environment on the well-being of migrant communities.

The next chapter, Chapter 2, sets the stage by further defining a critical approach and tackling important conceptual and terminological considerations. It begins from the perspective of critical border studies before examining ideas about migration and citizenship, embedded as they are in issues of sovereignty and legacies of colonialism. Next, it describes critical approaches to health, focusing on perspectives that privilege social determinants over individual behaviors.

Chapter 3 examines migrants' health in transit, focusing not solely on the journey itself but also the impacts of border control and immigration law in producing "illegality" for some populations. It frames impacts on health as necessarily located within the rise in the militarization of borders across the globe and the fundamental dilemma between demand for migrant labor and the lack of opportunities to cross borders legally. When people are compelled to migrate in an unauthorized manner, this results in specific and often violent risks to health, including death. Taking transit itself as a site of theoretical inquiry, it seeks to move the discussion beyond the binaries of push/pull factors and origin/destination countries to understand vulnerability, risk, and inequality. Forced immobility is a common pattern around the globe today, and so health is impacted not only by border crossings themselves but also by time spent waiting in border zones, refugee camps, migrant shelters, and detention centers. In addition, as a critical border studies perspective makes clear, borders themselves now frequently transcend physical space and reach into spaces of everyday life as strategic sites subject to intensified policing. Finally, this chapter examines the health impacts of family separation due to migration, as well as the positive and negative impacts of maintaining cross-border ties.

Chapter 4 explores the policy-level influences on migrant health, examining their impact on differential treatment and outcomes. Using a comparative approach, it examines the policy environment in various host nations (focusing primarily on undocumented or irregular migrants), illustrating how migrants are excluded from systems of health care promotion and provision. These policies create differential constructions of those seeking care and produce discourses of "deservingness," which frequently deem them unwanted, undesirable, and undeserving of protection or public support and ensuring continued marginalization. Even in purportedly universal health care systems, migrants are systematically excluded due to bureaucratic disentitlement and requirements to report their presence to authorities. There is a widespread disconnect between obligations under international rights conventions and how access to health care is translated in daily practice. As charities and humanitarian organizations step in to provide necessary services, their work can unintentionally legitimize shrinking public safety nets and tend to complicate the politics of care, create new forms of inequality. These efforts offer only short-term, improvisational solutions and can translate into absolving the state of its responsibilities. Finally, this chapter examines spillover effects on others, including family members and entire communities, whose well-being may be threatened by the combination of lack of health care access and pervasive fear of detention or deportation.

Chapter 5 critically explores the clinical encounter between migrants and the health care system – and the providers that work within them – in various receiving countries. It moves beyond questions of access to explore what happens in medical settings, ranging from public health departments, doctors' offices, and emergency rooms. Diverse populations create new challenges, and health systems and providers must adapt to meet these needs to avoid adverse outcomes for patients as well as systemic inefficiencies. This chapter illustrates how care is hampered by obstacles in the clinical environment, including cost, confusing organization of services, language barriers, different explanatory models of disease, perceived low quality of care, and social isolation. It argues for a move away from individual-based understandings and toward a focus on structural factors that are more likely to result in health inequalities. While cultural and language barriers between patients and clinicians are likely to lead to poor health outcomes, factors such as design of the health care system and a lack of understanding of migrants' everyday lives also play important roles. A critical perspective is necessary to focus on the systemic barriers to care and devise appropriate solutions, ranging from various forms of "competency" trainings and policies, increasing diversity in the clinical workforce, and building "migration aware" health systems.

Chapter 6 examines communicable disease and its relationship to human mobility, a topic which has become amplified in the wake of the recent pandemic. While patterns vary widely depending on the specific disease in question and are confounded by the heterogeneity of migrant populations, the linkage of migrants with infection – whether substantiated or not – offers important theoretical and practical insights from a critical perspective. This chapter uses three specific diseases – tuberculosis, HIV, and COVID-19 – to illustrate major themes: colonial legacies that have led to an association of migrants as diseased "others," resulting in persistent stigma for migrant communities; the strong association between communicable disease, relative deprivation, and social inequality; and political responses to outbreaks that involve limiting movement, border closures, and disproportionate impacts on marginalized populations. Negative perceptions of migrants also underlie border closures and other attempts to separate citizens from outsiders using emergency measures that are often unfounded in public health science. This highlights the perils of focusing on individual behavioral choices rather than on structural causes and systemic inequalities, and thus the importance of a critical perspective.

The search for work remains a principal driver of migration worldwide, and most migrants end up laboring in what have come to be known as "3-D jobs": dirty, demanding, and dangerous. Chapter 7 focuses on labor and occupational health since the robust link between mobility and the search for work influences all aspects of life. A critical approach is imperative, as race, ethnicity, nationality, gender, language, and legal status strongly determine the type of work people can access, and their vulnerability is amplified by exploitative labor arrangements. The environments in which migrants work are often substandard, endanger health, and increase risk for various forms of injury. On a global scale, they suffer from higher levels of occupational injury and fatality than native-born workers in the same sectors. At the same time, they lack access to adequate legal, social, and health care services and face coercion, fear, isolation, and racism. This chapter examines the dominant types of work that migrants perform in receiving societies and the health hazards associated with them, as well as constraints to seeking recourse. It focuses on the risks and injustices associated with immigrant labor, as well as the barriers to seeking medical care and worker compensation. The impact of workplace injuries and illnesses, it shows, reaches beyond the individual to affect families and broader communities. A critical perspective augments the scale of factors considered and employs the lenses of political economy and structural violence to understand how substandard conditions for injury and illness are produced.

The next chapter, Chapter 8, examines the impacts of gender and sexuality in the study of migrant health. It explores how migration policies are inscribed on bodies in ways that are gendered and gendering, in addition to intersecting with race and other factors. Gender is one of the fundamental social categories shaping immigration patterns today, producing major shifts in family structures, intimate relationships, and social roles. Sexuality is another important arena in which people contest and renegotiate the meanings behind citizenship and belonging (as well as "illegality") as it intersects with other relations of power related to race, gender, class, and geopolitics. The chapter includes a theoretical discussion of how migrant reproduction highlights notions of citizenship and belonging in host nations; reproduction is especially salient as it corresponds to various modes of citizenship with implications for conceptualization of migrant deservingness and access to services. Building upon the concept of "stratified reproduction," it explores how migrants' reproduction in host countries is a key feature of xenophobic fears of loss of a national identity or specific forms of "reconquest" or "demographic theft." This chapter also examines transnational parenting and caretaking in migrant families, and concludes by looking at the vulnerabilities and patterns associated with intimate partner violence. A critical approach is important to understand how structural and institutional violences impact experiences of sexuality, reproduction, family, parenting, and intimate relationships, often but not always deleteriously, because of migration, displacement, and separation.

Chapter 9 examines the health impacts of immigration enforcement, detention, and deportation. It illustrates how aggressive immigration regimes impact individual health behaviors and encourage discrimination. Enforcement policies and their subsequent actions – including arrest, detention, and deportation – perpetuate health disparities, exacerbate existing vulnerabilities related to legal status, and create new problems as they threaten the health and well-being of entire communities, including citizens. Intense surveillance, detention, and deportation have detrimental impacts on individual, family, and community health, disrupting social relationships and producing economic and psychosocial stressors. These frequently intersect with other vulnerabilities associated with poverty, racialization, and discrimination. Living with constant surveillance transforms public spaces into environments of risk, resulting in some people excluding themselves from certain health-promoting activities, places, and resources. Children whose parents have been deported experience a host of social disruptions and mental health problems. Assessing the complex relationship between immigration enforcement and health requires a critical perspective that emphasize systemic factors and the connection between social phenomena and political processes that produce poor health outcomes.

Refugee health is the subject of Chapter 10. Refugees and asylum seekers frequently inspire a different response in host communities than other forms of migrants based on notions of deservingness. While this opens some potential privileges, it still does not inoculate them from discrimination, obstacles to well-being, and overall poorer health outcomes. While refugees and asylum seekers may, under certain circumstances, have better access to state-sponsored services and welfare programs than other migrants fleeing less visible or less recognized forms of violence, the barriers to adequate health care and the benefits of full citizenship are still numerous. A unique characteristic of asylum seekers is their intimate contact with state governments, both in their home countries in the form of political violence and in receiving countries that decide which persons are "real" refugees through extensive processes of examination and surveillance. This chapter examines the complex relationship between state governments and health care regimes, illness origins and treatments within refugee populations, and claims of legitimacy.

Finally, the Conclusion summarizes major insights provided by a critical perspective, proposed areas of intervention, and explicates future research needs and strategies to tackle the health inequities that affect migrants.

2

CRITICAL PERSPECTIVES ON MIGRATION AND HEALTH

A critical perspective on migration and health requires an interdisciplinary set of ideas about borders, sovereignty, mobilities, citizenship, race, and various forms of systemic violence that affect health at the collective, rather than solely individual, level. This chapter further defines this framework and introduces theoretical concepts employed in the remainder of the book, all of which have important epistemological and analytical implications for understanding migrant health. It begins from the perspective of critical border studies, which decenters borders as taken-for-granted entities and treats them as sites in a constant process of becoming. Bordering, here, refers to a variety of everyday inclusionary and exclusionary practices, creating "internal" boundaries in addition to those physical boundaries located at the edges of state territory. The chapter then turns to ideas about migration and citizenship, embedded as they are in issues of sovereignty and legacies of colonialism, and seeks to trouble commonly held assumptions about the boundary between the two categories. Next, it moves to describe a variety of critical approaches to health, calling especially for an understanding of the social determinants of health over approaches that foreground individual behaviors. A critical framing focuses on the social origins of illness and disease, and especially on the context that produces them, to explain how inequality, poverty, institutional constraints, and violence contribute to health disparities.

Critical Border Studies

Borders have a seductive charm. They offer a sense of certainty and security, even as we repeatedly witness their contingent and indeterminate character (Parker & Vaughan-Williams 2009). Rather than simply being proverbial "lines in the sand" that divide territories, borders are complex social, political, and cultural processes and discourses (Johnson et al. 2011) that require attention to the inclusionary

DOI: 10.4324/9781003307532-2

and exclusionary practices associated with them. There is a long tradition of critical theoretical insights about borders in contemporary political life, primarily in reconceptualizing what is commonly understood to be "the razor-edge of the nation-state where mutually recognised sovereignties meet and yet do not overlap" (Parker & Vaughan-Williams 2012: 728). Alongside this, the new mobilities turn in the social sciences has challenged the sedentist framing that "treats as normal stability, meaning, and place, and treats as abnormal distance, change, and placelessness" (Sheller & Urry 2006: 209). This has led to a rejection of approaches that rely on conceptions of territorial nationalism in understanding migration and mobilities more broadly.

One fundamental goal of a critical approach is thus to denaturalize the concept of borders as a reified object. Borders do not only exist as marks on a map but are continually shifting and (re)emerging. They are processes rather than static things, always in the process of becoming. They are brought into being through performances, that is, through rituals such as passport inspections or customs procedures (Parker & Vaughan-Williams 2012).

A related point is that the relationship between borders and (sovereign) territory has become ever more complex (Parker & Vaughan-Williams 2009). The concept of the nation-state as some sort of neat and tidy "container-box" has never been accurate, with critical scholars pointing to the "territorial trap" – that is, the fallacy that there is a fixed, absolute spatial ordering of sovereign territory, or a perfect alignment between the geography and the political (Gielis & van Houtum 2012). Today, bordering practices are increasingly intangible or ephemeral, pushing beyond territorial logic to include electronic technologies and tracking data, for example.

At the same time, this does not mean that the salience of borders has gone away. Borders persist in defining insiders and outsiders and producing violence for some groups over others. They are certainly not the same everywhere for everyone; while some border crossers are labeled "unauthorized" or "illegal," others become "trusted travelers," whose "customer experience" is of highest priority. Recognition of this unequal landscape of border experiences is the foundation of the argument made here.

This book joins other scholars in calling for a concerted effort to "decenter," trouble, destabilize, or unsettle the border, that is, problematize it as a taken-for-granted object when in fact it is always shifting, becoming, and being performed. This perspective allows for the exploration of alternative border epistemologies and imaginaries (Parker & Vaughan-Williams 2012). A critical approach can highlight the shifting reality of borders, as well as

> determining the associations between that and our broader spatial and governmental imaginaries; subjecting border-making practices to critical scrutiny; evaluating the ethical and political aspects of border regimes and control; and thus, finally, setting the study of "the border", its cognates, and border-studies own research agenda in a self-critical light.
>
> *Parker & Vaughan-Williams 2009: 583*

One epistemic corrective that results from this perspective is the rejection of clean binary oppositions which borders appear to present. Instead, we are encouraged to consider alternative objects, metaphors, and vocabularies focused less on inside/outside or citizen/foreigner (or citizen/migrant) and instead examine situations and spaces that are thresholds or in-between. This also requires us to rethink border spatialities with questions such as "How do borders open/foreclose different possibilities? What does it mean to transgress a border (e.g., in 'illegal' migration) and how does transgression produce the very border that is seemingly transgressed?" as well as border temporalities: "How do borders change? What is the 'time-print' of the border? How do pre-emptive practices such as are characteristic of EU enlargement, globalisation, etc disrupt the familiar temporal registers within which borders have been conceptualised?" (see Parker & Vaughan-Williams 2009: 585).

A final epistemic corrective is to approach borders as phenomenological events, that is, as objects that are experienced by people as opposed to fixed realities. Here, we must ask questions such as, "How do people experience border-crossing? What does it feel like to exist as a border, as unwelcome migrants are forced to do? To what extent are border experiences determined by national and/or racial predicates" (Parker & Vaughan-Williams 2009)?

"Citizens" and "Migrants": Questions of Sovereignty, Il/Legality, and Inequality

The study of migration is ultimately also a study of citizenship. Citizenship represents the most visible example of state power and sovereignty as the underlying legal capacity to create forms of difference, resulting from broader engagements with globalization and colonialism. The unsettling of sovereignty helps to highlight the persistence of colonial power (Bonilla 2017; Mbembé 2003); in a world increasingly composed of populations displaced by these global forces, nation-states continue to define themselves in relationship to entities defined as Other, reinforcing the ability to "legislate, deport, invade, build and borrow." One of the paradoxes of modernity is that the number of humans without a sovereign nation – refugees, exiled minorities, internally displaced persons – continue to grow at the same time as states double down on sovereign claims, borders, boundaries, and bans. Those left outside the nation-state are dehumanized – living in non-sovereign states with minimal political life – floating in a state of exception with no specific legal status (Bonilla 2017).

One could argue that citizenship is about the "lottery of birth" or, more precisely, the passport one holds. The opportunity to migrate, especially in terms of visa access, varies greatly around the globe, and there is even a global ranking of countries according to the mobility freedom of their citizens (the Henley Passport Index). Citizens from countries with "very high levels of human development" can travel visa-free to around 85% of all other countries worldwide (IOM 2022). Notably, these are generally the same countries that are preferred destinations for international migrants. On the other hand, visa restrictions are in place for nationals from countries with "very low levels of human development," thus closing off migration pathways and making irregular opportunities to be the only – or certainly the most realistic – option to them.

From a critical perspective, ease of migration is not simply a result of the "lottery of birth" but a major and intentional feature of unequal global relations rooted in colonialism. Visa access, and the freedom of movement that accompanies it, is a clear measure of a country's status within the global community. Immigration law and practices such as visa access and opportunities for regularization are highly structured by a system of preferences. In some place, these preferences are related to labor market needs or reserved for those with high degrees of human or economic capital. In others, preferences hinge on having specific family ties, as is the case in the U.S. Individuals have little chance of becoming legal immigrants without evidence of belonging in one of these preference categories, regardless of personal qualities such as being hardworking, highly educated, or law-abiding. Finally, admission via the mechanisms of political asylum and refugee status are reserved for only a select few.

Critical scholarship on migration has particularly focused on "illegality" – that is, uncertain legal status, or living as a migrant "without papers" or without a valid residency permit – and its impacts on experiences of well-being. The condition of "illegality" here refers to a sociopolitical condition, juridical status, and relationship to the state (De Genova 2002; Inda 2006; Ngai 2014). The choice of terminology for this condition is highly varied, including illegal, undocumented, irregular, extra-legal, unauthorized, or clandestine, as well as terms such as *sans papiers* in French, *sin papeles* in Spanish, and *ohne Papiere* in German – all of which are precise in their own ways and in particular contexts. Additionally, this concept may refer to a variety of circumstances, such as illegal entry into a country, illegal residency following legal entry (that is, overstaying the duration of a visa), or illegal employment. In other cases, newly rearranged state boundaries may exclude already resident groups as legitimately belonging, essentially "erasing" former identities, as happened in the former Yugoslavia.

While some have stressed that use of the term "illegal" implies collusion with particular hegemonic constructions, other scholars have advocated retaining the term precisely to further explore this sociojuridical status. They argue that employing the term allows us to (1) deconstruct it as the object of study itself, (2) emphasize the legal context that provides form and content to the everyday lives of migrants, and (3) investigate how this construction implicitly places migrants outside the scope and protection of the rule of law (Willen 2007). Put another way, people are not "illegal," but they can become "illegalized" through their particular relationship with a state and its practices.

Nonetheless, attentiveness to the condition of "illegality" must not result in framing people as passive subjects with a homogeneous set of experiences, since people always also adapt their daily lives and develop strategies in response to the circumstances of their precarious lives. Attentiveness to "illegality" does not mean constructing people as "passive and agency-less subjects overdetermined by structural conditions, or undocumentedness as a homogeneous and undifferentiated experience" (Sigona 2012: 51).

"Deportation regimes" around the world further work to produce individuals' prolonged susceptibility to being deported (De Genova 2002), which is more effective than the presumed deterrance functions of a militarized border alone or the impact of restrictive immigration policies. Interrelated systems of immigration control – external/territorial and internal/social – construct migrants as a racialized Other, reinforcing ideas of illegality while undermining it when it benefits particular economic and political interests (Fassin 2011). Deportability ensures that irregular or undocumented labor is rendered a uniquely disposible commodity (De Genova 2002; Peutz & De Genova 2010), which has implications for well-being as well as heightened risk of injury and illness.

In recent years, the concept of *precarity* has emerged to describe the multiple forms of dispossession that some populations face as part of increased economic uncertainty, violence, political marginalization, and injustice. Precarity is not simply a condition, but a process built into institutions to create a heightened sense of expendability or disposability for some groups in society. In the case of vulnerable legal status, this state of permanent vulnerability and precaritization translates directly into deportability (Armenta 2017; De Genova 2002, 2016; Golash-Boza 2015; Gomberg-Munoz & Nussbaum-Barberena 2011; Schierup & Jørgensen 2017). In relation to health, precarity is understood as increased physical and emotional vulnerability, exposure to risk, instability, and lack of recourse in the face of access barriers and injustices.

In migration studies, precarity is also visible in the practices of granting temporary legal status, temporary residence permits, or deferred deportation. There has been a policy shift around the globe that has led to a proliferation of provisional, interim, temporary, and precarious statuses (Abrego & Lakhani 2015; Coutin et al. 2017; Landolt & Goldring 2016; Menjívar 2014; Menjívar & Kanstroom 2013). These forms of "liminal" or temporary legality are intended to prevent long-term settlement and offer no opportunities for permanency. This produces a persistent vulnerability and insecurity, along with "new and pernicious forms of inequality" (Gomberg-Muñoz 2016: 5). These programs frequently entail a shift from random encounters with the state and institutions of immigration enforcement to routine but indefinite surveillance. As a result, people become documented, yet remain deportable; they are recognized by the state, but never truly authorized. Scholars have described these experiences as "spaces of nonexistence" (Coutin 2000), in which people are physically and socially present but without legal status. As a result of their altered yet persistent condition of illegality, their lives become full of uncertainty and everyday anxieties, as well as direct institutional violence and discrimination.

Managing migration, thus, is both a reflection of and mechanism for national sovereignty (De Genova 2002; Inda 2006; Nevins 2001; Ngai 2014). In studying "migrants," it is important to first, understand and, second, avoid reinscribing the global inequalities that produce people who cross state borders as non-citizen "outsiders" or "foreigners" (De Genova 2016). To truly approach the topic with a critical lens, one must begin with the concept of citizenship to theorize migration both with an eye toward the "the transnational class politics of human mobility, which routinely transposes a global relation of capital and labor into the ostensibly insular statist ('national') politics of 'immigration' and border policing" (De Genova 2016: 236), in addition to "global postcolonial politics of race that reactivates and refortifies 'national' (or supranational) state borders as so many 'color lines', which nevertheless may be seen as often as not to dissimulate race in favor of a nativist politics of citizenship" (De Genova 2016: 236). As a result, some have argued that a critical approach must "take as its first premise the priority and prerogative of the elemental and elementary human freedom of movement" (De Genova 2016: 236). The implication here is clear: to recognize that migration is not fundamentally transgressive, exceptional, or pathological.

Another major proposition is that analyses must avoid implicitly placing Western/Northern countries as the only, primary, or preferred destinations in the migrant imagination. Postcolonial approaches offer a correction here, as they seek to debunk "conventional dichotomous, and essentially colonial, ways of conceptualizing global migration" (Berriane et al. 2015: 517). Studies that are theorized from the epistemic perspective of the migrant-receiving country exemplify this bias. This also has important consequences for researcher positionality, as it is frequently coupled with the unproblematized viewpoint of those who authorize themselves to speak for the citizens of the migrant-receiving nation-state (De Genova 2016). In other words, the researcher's positionality is "significantly substantiated in his/her juridical status as citizen, and so entails a social relation to the state; as such, it is an eminently *political* identity, indeed a *bordered* identity" (De Genova 2016: 230, italics in original). To avoid uncritical ethnocentrism, we must avoid thinking about migration from the implicit perspective of citizens; in other words, we should not take for granted our own position as part of the inequality intrinsic to citizenship itself.

Who Is a Migrant? Conceptual Pitfalls

There are several linguistic and conceptual pitfalls common in the study of migrant health. Terminology matters a great deal in shaping how the topic is discussed, and this framing also impacts how migrants are received by a host country. Who is an im/migrant? What are the different forms of migration and mobility? Why is terminology so critical?

Throughout the book, I make an effort to utilize the term "migrant" rather than *immigrant* to avoid implying the unilinear teleology of categories (De Genova 2002), since the term "immigrant" is implicitly positioned from the perspective of "receiving" societies. However, because the discussions are drawn from a variety of scholarship, representing different fields and conventions, this cannot always be consistent, and I often utilize the terminology employed by the original researchers whose work I cite. Similarly, other terms (e.g., "host" vs. "receiving" countries) are used interchangeably for this reason. Nonetheless, an awareness of the implications of these choices must be made clear up front.

While definitions of migrant status vary substantially, the IOM defines a migrant as,

> An umbrella term, not defined under international law, reflecting the common lay understanding of a person who moves away from his or her place of usual residence, whether within a country or across an international border, temporarily or permanently, and for a variety of reasons.
>
> *IOM 2019:* 132

In other words, this term encompasses a variety of legal categories including migrant workers, particular types of movements, such as smuggled persons, as well as persons whose movements are not specifically defined under international law, including students.

However, migration is not a singular activity but involves a complex set of variables, including different forms of entry and legal status (permanent legal resident, temporary work visa, undocumented), different intentions of settlement (permanent vs. temporary), temporal mobility patterns (seasonal movement vs. continued residence in a single location). As a result, there is a variety of definitions across existing scholarship. It is further important to recognize the intersectional nature of the migrant experience with regards to sociodemographic factors (e.g., gender, race, national origin, sexual orientation) in addition to varied experiences across the life course. This allows for critical insight into processes that "create and reinforce indicators of social stratification, and the ways that health-related opportunities as well as injustices and inequalities are enacted on a multidimensional basis" (Thomas 2016: 5).

Processes of illegalization are another important feature of contemporary migration and play an important role in this book. These processes are directly linked to other histories of colonialism, slavery, genocide, settlement, and annexation in the making of nation-states around the globe. In recent decades, there has been an increasing emphasis on the legality of migrants, including its impacts for health and wellbeing, so this is a major focus of the book. Il/legal status is understood to be rooted in historical processes that designate migrant populations as "legal" or "illegal," "regular" or "irregular," so that these categories are constructions and in fact contingent, unstable, and the outcome of multiple relations of power (Luibhéid 2008: 289). Since it is a sociolegal construction, dependent on laws and context, people who are legal immigrants can become illegal, and vice versa, and these various constructions have changed over time. For example, the idea of the "illegal alien" in the United States (U.S.) was historically constructed through a combination of exclusionary immigration laws and the creation of the Border Patrol in 1924, without existing as a concept beforehand.

Another important consideration is, Who is considered a refugee? According to the 1951 Convention relating to the Status of Refugees, a refugee is someone who, "owing to a well-founded fear of persecution for reasons of race, religion, nationality, membership of a particular social group or political opinion, is outside the country of his nationality and is unable or, owing to such fear, is unwilling to avail himself of the protection of that country" (IOM 2019: 132); furthermore, it includes those "who, not having a nationality and being outside the country of his former habitual residence as a result of such events, is unable or, owing to such fear, is unwilling to return to it" (IOM 2019: 132). But is only someone facing political persecution a "true" refugee, in contrast to those seeking economic opportunity? Our common usage of this term often defies the official definition. In addition, some advocate eliminating the distinction between "economic" and "political" refugees to highlight the causes of displacement globally, especially national and supranational economic policies, through an explicitly anticolonial perspective (Wright 2003). At the same time, it is important to consider the impacts of conflating refugees and asylum seekers with other kinds of migrants. First, the indiscriminate use of the term "refugee" can further delegitimize the unique forms of suffering for those who experienced forced migration due to political violence. Second, while highlighting the role of structural economic violence, this can obscure the fact that refugees and asylum seekers generally are perceived as "more deserving" and often have limited but guaranteed access to health care, in contrast to unauthorized persons. This distinction is crucial in understanding the distribution of rights and resources, an important point of this book. Health outcomes across migrant groups vary by route of entry, affecting experiences during the immigration process and degrees of access to health services in the receiving country after arrival (Giuntella et al. 2018).

One of the most pressing issues in the world today, migration is frequently referred to as a "crisis." This alarmist framing often provokes extreme political responses and sensationalist media attention. Over the last decade, for instance, the European Union (EU) has received incomparable numbers of migrants, asylum seekers, and refugees, leading some to describe it as a "global migration magnet" (Czaika & Haas 2014). In other countries, like the U.S., people speak of a "surge" or "flood" of migrants entering the country, especially via the southern border with Mexico. In the media and in politics, we hear of migration from Africa, the Middle East, and Latin America not infrequently described as "swarms," "hordes," and "marauders," and this is not coincidentally occurring at the same time as the rise of isolationist nationalism in many places, including the U.S., Britain, Netherlands, Austria, Poland, Italy, and Germany (Holmes & Castañeda 2016; Lee et al. 2018). These framings serve to produce public and political anxiety as well as regular "border spectacles" (De Genova 2013). A critical approach rejects the use of violent and militarized terms such as "crisis," or "floods," as well as dehumanizing language such as "illegal immigrant" or "unaccompanied alien minor."

Migration is of course deeply racialized, alongside conceptions of belonging, otherness, and citizenship. Migration status is frequently conflated with other forms of difference, especially for communities of color (e.g., those inhabited by racial or ethnic minorities). Despite living there for generations, in some countries, ethnic, religious, or tribal groups are still perceived to be "foreign" (even "migrant") communities (Lee et al. 2018). The children of migrants have long held a tenuous place in various countries and are often racialized in a way that they are characterized as perpetual foreigners, even if they are citizens, since whiteness is frequently the unspoken master narrative about citizenship and belonging. In the U.S., for instance, citizen children of im/migrants have been derided as "anchor babies" or treated as "suspect citizens" (Chavez 2017), constructed as a racial threat to the nation. Young U.S.-born Latinos may experience belonging as "citizens, but not Americans" (Flores-González 2017). Their everyday experiences, including spatial segregation, microaggressions, and anti-Latino rhetoric, belie their status as citizens, underscoring the persistent role of race in notions of belonging to this imagined community. People may thus be treated as "alien citizens" – that is, citizens by birth but whose migrant ancestry renders their status as citizens dubious – as they are cast as perpetual foreigners (Ngai 2014). In Germany, second-, third-, and even fourth-generation individuals born in Germany but with Turkish heritage experience similar exclusions. The categories used to differentiate between groups of people often reproduce "othering" discourses and can complicate a thorough analysis of health inequalities or access barriers (Wenner et al. 2019). On the other hand, there exists wide variation in different countries. For example, in the United Arab Emirates, over 88% of the population are international migrants (IOM 2022).

In sum, legitimacy depends on changing and historically produced notions of relative deservingness that emulates distinctions made between citizens and various kinds of "others" in different national settings (Willen 2010). Thus, it is important to ask: when does a migrant cease to be a migrant and become a "native," or a "citizen"? what about descendants of the enslaved in places like the Americas? Are they considered migrants, and why or why not? At what point do they cease to be, or does exclusion just take on different conceptual forms over time? These questions highlight the often artificial boundaries set within notions of relative belonging, since even "natives" or "citizens" may be socially cast as foreigners, particularly if they or their family have any migrant background at all. In addition, in many places we are seeing the rise of mixed-status families, which contain varied constellations of citizens, permanent legal residents, undocumented migrants, and individuals in legal limbo. All this is to say that it is not facile to draw lines between migrant and non-migrant populations, and the disparities they may experience in the forms of inequality, poverty, and institutional constraints still impact health.

Understandably, most scholarly approaches to migration (and especially migrant health) presume that migrants are disadvantaged in comparison to citizens of the host country. However, we must also acknowledge that not all migrants are poor, disadvantaged, or the targets of discrimination. In many cases – and for a variety of reasons including dissonance of health understandings or distrust with an unfamiliar health care system – migrants maintain ties and engage with systems and care practices in their country of origin. For instance, Korean migrants to New Zealand may travel to their homeland to obtain medical procedures, based on preferences for decisive and comprehensive treatment in culturally comfortable settings (Lee et al. 2010). Similarly, Mexican migrants in the U.S. are often able to cross the border and use their earnings to visit private doctors and clinics in Mexico. These medical returns not only provide them access to care that is familiar and viewed as more effective but also enabled class transformation, as migrants transitioned from poor rural peasants to cash-paying "returning royalty" in their home country (Horton 2014).

Finally, it is imperative to remember that the term "migrant" represents an identity imposed from the outside – by the researcher, the media, politicians, or society at large. Many people identify first and foremost with other characteristics of their lives as lived daily: mother, daughter, student, artist, engineer, Muslim, neighbor, and so on. By considering their primary point of reference to be migration status, we create and endorse superficial and reductive identities and perpetuate narratives that reinforce social barriers.

Critical Perspectives on Health

Critical perspectives on health have their roots in the tradition of social medicine. Developed in the wake of the industrial revolution in response to increased levels of disease and poverty among workers, social medicine focuses on the socioeconomic conditions affecting health, illness, and the practice of medicine. This book takes a critical framing by focusing on the these origins of illness, and particularly how inequality, poverty, institutional constraints, and violence contribute to produce health disparities in some populations.

Migration itself does not create risks to health; certain vulnerabilities must first exist. Framing migration as a public health issue may be a bold claim for those who espouse a narrow view of the prevention of disease (Wild & Dawson 2018). However, this book takes a broader approach to examine the structural factors determined by social and economic policies and institutional contexts that foster unequal effects on health. This critical approach emerges from larger theoretical traditions in the social sciences and is located within a set of broader frameworks and concepts for understanding the effects of social inequality. This perspective challenges us to interrogate assumptions, understand what is socially constructed, and be more precise about how we define the impacts of immigration on health as opposed to using migration status as a proxy for other social dynamics, such as inequality, marginalization, or race. These impacts must also be understood as intersectional, since health-related injustices and inequalities are enacted on a multidimensional basis dependent on factors such as gender, age, country of origin, sexual orientation, and social class (Thomas 2016).

Several fields have related theories, models, frameworks, and vocabulary that highlight these issues. For instance, critical public health approaches include a range of overlapping concepts for understanding and responding to the effects of social inequality, including *social epidemiology*, the *eco-social* or *socio-environmental perspective*, *eco-epidemiology*, and the *risk environment framework*. A focus on social inequalities can be explored through *fundamental social causes*, *social determinants of health*, *webs of causation*, *higher-order causal-level structural factors*, *upstream factors*, and *racial disparities in health outcomes*. The social sciences have contributed frameworks using *political economy*, *structural violence*, *symbolic violence*, *structural vulnerability*, *syndemic vulnerability*, *conjugated oppression*, *hierarchies of embodied suffering*, *zones of abandonment*, *intersectionality*, and *discourses of deservingness*. These approaches all emphasize the influence of social structures and the relative positions of groups within stratified hierarchies and power relationships.

Many of these concepts have influenced and/or emerged from models that focus on the *social determinants of health*, useful for examining health in migrant populations and for guiding population-level interventions. Social determinants of health refer to the contexts that produce ill health and health disparities, which may include legal status, language barriers, institutional racism, trauma associated with migration, obstacles to accessing medical care, the lack of legal or civil protections, and occupational hazards. Attending to these structural issues is often an important consideration for understanding illness beyond the observable biopathogenic processes and can lead to policy and health-system changes to improve outcomes (Dubal et al. 2021). The analysis of disease causation, as well as intervention strategies and policy changes to address it, requires an understanding of how social, physical, and biological phenomena interrelate and overlap. As a result, pathways and interactions are understood as multicausal and complex, requiring attention to institutional practices and to the relationships between macrostructural processes and microlevel behaviors.

Although migration is a consequence of social determinants, such as poverty, educational opportunities, and/or political persecution, migration must also be positioned as a social determinant in its own right (Castañeda et al. 2015). Without this perspective, the experience is cast as secondary to more proximal factors such as behavior, language, norms, income, or education, thus limiting explanatory power and the capacity to create effective interventions that respond to some of the root causes of ill-health in communities. The vast consequences of immigration on everyday life, and thus on broader health and well-being, cannot be reduced simply to a "protective factor" or an acculturative "stressor." Rather, immigration itself must be understood as a social determinant of health and well-being. Examining it through this lens provides a more holistic understanding of these complex, interrelated, and far-reaching impacts. A narrow focus on "risk factors" and behavioral or cultural modifications uncritically assumes the unfettered agency of marginalized populations (e.g., Castañeda et al. 2015; Quesada et al. 2011). Responding to individualistic, non-contextualized approaches to explaining this distribution of adverse health outcomes, a critical approach argues for the examination of the role of social inequality, which imposes specific risks and constraints on choice. (e.g., Krieger 2013, 2016; Lupton 1999, 2000). Critical approaches thus provide a corrective for superficial notions of individual behavioral and cultural difference that rest on static assumptions about migration choice, intergroup relations, and unidirectional advantages of assimilation.

Put another way, a critical approach interprets health outcomes by understanding and accounting for the large-scale structures that impact them. Throughout the book, several concepts are employed to illuminate these factors. *Structural violence* is utilized by scholars in fields such as medical anthropology, medical sociology, and social epidemiology to explain the processes by which the arrangement of social institutions causes harm by depriving people of resources or preventing them from reaching their potential (Farmer 2001). It is particularly useful for explaining differential health outcomes among populations as they relate to broader, macrolevel social forces. These arrangements are structural because they are

> embedded in the political and economic organization of our social world; they are violent because they cause injury to people … neither culture nor pure individual will is at fault; rather, historically given (and often economically driven) processes and forces conspire to constrain individual agency.
>
> *Farmer 2001: 79*

Yet while this concept recognizes the complex web of social, political, and economic forces that constrain individual and community health, structural violence can also be ambiguous, making it difficult to operationalize interventions and address the "social machinery of oppression" (Rodgers and O'Neill 2012; see also Dubal et al. 2021).

Structural vulnerability is an extension of this concept that focuses on relative location in a hierarchical social order defined by the intersection of these larger structural forces (Quesada et al. 2011). This location produces increased suffering and risk for certain diseases, reduced access to care, and poor health outcomes, as such positioning is derived from "forces that constrain decision making, frame choices, and limit life options" (Quesada et al. 2011: 341–342). Another useful concept here is that of *syndemics*, which highlights mutually reinforcing sets of health, environmental, and social challenges encountered by marginalized populations (Alexander & Fernandez 2014; Singer & Clair 2003). This concept recognizes the

> fundamental biosocial nature of health and the ways that diseases and other health-related conditions interact synergistically, in consequential and often deleterious ways … emphasizes the ways that social conditions and relationships shape disease processes, including contagion, through political-economic, structural, and environmental factors.
>
> *Singer & Rylko-Bauer 2021: 8–9*

For example, diabetes has been examined as a syndemic because of its comorbidity with HIV in Kenya, tuberculosis in India, and depression in South Africa. The concept highlights interactions between pathophysiology, the structure of health care systems, socioeconomic conditions, and cultural context (Mendenhall et al. 2017). These processes of power exhibit strong influence over the life chances of migrants and their families, creating obstacles to well-being and health care access.

Another related perspective focuses on *infrastructural determinants of health*, which examines larger historical and political frameworks that determine the social determinants (Dubal et al. 2021). These include race, political economy, history, and borders themselves, all of which underlie experiences of health and illness. Drawing on the notion of infrastructural violence (Rodgers & O'Neill 2012), this approach aims to confront and transform "an enormous set of colonizing, racist hegemonic assumptions and ways of thinking – a project necessary in truly revolutionizing the ways in which migrant illness is approached and treated" (Dubal et al. 2021: 2). It reframes the issue to focus on "the lasting material channels," including borders themselves as both physical and ideological infrastructure. This approach examines the complex histories of inequalities by examining their even deeper historical and political roots. An illustrative example, to use the case of Central American migrants coming to the U.S., includes the "plans, histories, policies, and peoples involved in building the conditions for migration … including forces of colonialism, U.S. imperialism, neoliberalism, and border militarization" (Dubal et al. 2021: 1). Thus, structural violence is in many ways the outcome of decades of U.S. involvement, which has focused extractionist policies and military interference in the region. A historically attentive approach can shift discourse to respond in different and more radical ways beyond short-term and often misplaced humanitarian efforts.

Indeed, a major argument of this book is that assumptions regarding root causes of migration shape ideas about how deserving (of incorporation, health, wellness, or flourishing) a particular migrant group is. Here, the concept of *deservingness* can aid in understanding its implications for health (Willen 2010). Migrant deservingness both shapes and reflects policies of entitlement and exclusion; as such, the legal entitlements for certain groups can also shape how the public perceives and portrays their collective deservingness, including their access to and quality of health care. Constantly shifting and historically produced notions of how deserving a group is in comparison to other groups pits them against each other in a hierarchy of legitimacy in the face of scarce resources. For example, a refugee who has fled violence in their home country may be viewed as more "deserving" of time and resources in the clinical setting than an undocumented migrant laborer. As migrants are generally excluded to some extent from systems of health care promotion and provision, differential constructions of deservingness deem them unwanted, undesirable, and undeserving of protection or support and ensuring continued marginalization. Migrant wellbeing is thus the result of policies of both exclusion and entitlement, which shape health through inherent risk and access to care (Sargent 2012).

Deservingness effects on differential access to health care is also inherently linked to concepts of humanitarianism and human rights. Market-based health care has led to a proliferation of non-governmental organizations (NGOs) providing health care to migrants and other underserved populations. Critical approaches are wary of humanitarian discourse that overfocuses on subjects' suffering (or trauma) at the expense of structural cause and solutions. Humanitarianism is rooted in particular ideas of deservingness that migrants and refugees must work hard to establish and is further flawed in its assumption that any help is better than nothing (Ticktin 2014). Moreover, these solutions that arise within humanitarian spaces that are often steeped in deficit thinking, seeking only to educate or provide resources so that structural barriers can be overcome rather than explicitly challenged.

"Healthy Migrant Effects" and Immigrant Health Paradoxes

So, how do these critical approaches fit into conventional ways of understanding the relationship between migration and health? The following sections cover some major acknowledged patterns – healthy migrant effects, migrant health paradoxes, and the health impacts of assimilation, incorporation, and acculturation – and discusses their relationship to critical approaches.

Decades ago, researchers identified a significant pattern among migrant groups: their mortality rates were frequently lower compared to local (native) populations. In general, it does hold true that migrants are less likely than their non-migrant peers to report a chronic health problem, defined as persisting one year or longer (Giuntella et al. 2018). The concept of the "healthy migrant effect" was developed to explain this phenomenon, positing that since most migrants are seeking work opportunities, only people of good general health choose to, are chosen to, or are able to migrate. In other words, some amount of self-selection is at work, which ultimately impacts health status. Research further suggests that migrants arrive with healthier diets and lifestyles than their peers, which make them – at least initially – to be less susceptible for chronic illnesses.

However, the picture is much more complex than this. First, while much evidence supports the healthy migrant effect, there remain issues with establishing causality (Lu & Zhang 2016). Earlier studies on the healthy migrant effect often carried inherent biases because of their selective focus on cardiovascular diseases. Critiques of this approach (Spallek et al. 2016) note that research needs to (1) better account for the heterogeneity of migrant populations, (2) attend to macrolevel social determinants that influence health outcomes in the host country, and that (3) a life-course approach is best suited to capture the temporal dimensions of exposures and risk accumulation over time.

Even when immigrants are healthier on arrival, their purpose for migrating and support networks play an important role in their overall health. A UK-based study found significant differences by reason for migration, with those migrating for employment, family reunification, or higher education reporting better health outcomes compared to asylum seekers and refugees (Giuntella et al. 2018). In addition, prolonged separation from family members across international borders negatively impacts health and incorporation experiences. For example, research has found a significant association between family separation and poorer health among sub-Saharan African immigrant women in France (Afulani et al. 2016).

Finally, and perhaps most notably, research increasingly also shows that migrants' health quickly and markedly deteriorates after arrival in a host country (Gushulak

2007; Woodward et al. 2014). While recent immigrants may have a health advantage, the longer they live in a host country, the poorer their health status becomes (Antecol & Bedard 2006; Fennelly 2007). Studies in multiple settings have found that health status converges to that of natives over time, or may become worse on average.

Although social exclusion and economic marginalization associated with migration status often declines over time and for each subsequent generation through processes of incorporation, there is contradictory evidence regarding effects on health. In many cases, researchers have noted that migrants who are less assimilated (or "acculturated") appear to exhibit better health outcomes than more assimilated or native-born individuals. This "immigrant health paradox" has been explored extensively in the U.S., especially with migrants of Latin American and Asian origin, but with inconsistent and equivocal findings. Studies of health behaviors and risk factor profiles among Latinx populations, for example, show that greater acculturation is associated with increased alcohol intake, smoking, and high body mass index (BMI; Abraído-Lanza et al. 2005). In addition, rates of specific cancer as well as diet-related diseases (cardiovascular disease, gall bladder disease) are generally lower among Latinx populations but tend to converge over time as they become more acculturated (Lara et al. 2005).

Since there is robust evidence that the health status of immigrants deteriorates after a certain time in a host country, researchers frequently view a lack of acculturation or assimilation as the underlying mechanism. However, these concepts too have been faulted for their underlying assumptions and lack of accounting for structural factors, as the following section elaborates.

Integration, Incorporation, and Acculturation

Critiques of acculturation studies have underscored the vagueness and bias associated with this concept, focused on their largely unexplored underlying assumptions. First, they presume that immigrants enjoy some collection of cultural features or habits that predispose them to better health status. Health outcomes (whether positive, negative, or neutral) among minority groups is routinely attributed to "freewheeling applications of culture" (Hunt & DeVoogd 2005) that lack specificity. While several methods and scales have been developed to measure the advantages of acculturation or assimilation of immigrants into a host society, they often fail to explicitly define what is being described. For instance, health researchers may attribute mental health status to the protective effect of "traditional culture retention" (Escobar & Vega 2000) without specifying what that is, or the combination of "culturally based fatalistic attitudes" and cumulative negative life experiences (Ruef et al. 2000). The basis for comparison is sketchy at best; instead of a thorough examination of context, it is assumed that correlation implies causation, and many variables are left undefined or unexplored.

Second, studies rely on superficial and stereotyped notions of "culture." As a result, acculturation scales present a static view of intergroup relations and a belief that this process is uniform across populations. Latinos, for example, are largely viewed as a homogeneous group, instead of accounting for different histories and contexts of migration, class, and the presence of large native U.S. Latinx population (and U.S.-born native Latinx are often used as a comparison group based on implicit but very problematic notions of genetic or heritable relatedness). Change in cultural habits is not viewed as potentially reciprocal – most scales typically only measure unidirectional change – and is generally viewed as inevitable over time.

Third, most acculturation studies carry the tacit assumption that health care services and overall quality of life in the host country are incommensurably better than those found in the country of origin (Jass and Massey 2004). Related to this, these approaches generally do not measure comparative data on local (native) populations. Acculturation studies rarely explore previous living conditions or habits in the country of origin, thus excluding important information about health status over the life course and in different environments. While the issue of pre-migration stressors and living conditions has received some attention (Himmelgreen et al. 2007; Thurston & Vissandjée 2005), solid analyses is required to prevent stereotyping of cultural difference (Hunt et al. 2004).

Put another way, these approaches are often reductionist and exclude structural factors that could contribute to the deteriorating health of immigrants over time, such as inaccessible health care, lack of resources, or inadequate communication with health providers (Cristancho et al. 2008). Furthermore, a narrow focus on cultural behaviors or sets of risk factors unique to specific groups "uncritically assumes the unfettered agency of vulnerable populations, endowing their behaviors with a misplaced sense of autonomy" (Horton 2016: 4). An individualistic, non-contextualized approach to explaining adverse health outcomes fails to recognize how these are unevenly distributed in ways that disproportionately impact the health and well-being of immigrants, women, and working people of color. Intersectionality is one correctional lens that allows us to challenge such overgeneralizations – not all migrants experience health and illness in the same way – and include the effects of gender, race, class, ethnicity, country of origin, and so forth. Racial and gender ideologies and discourse interact with migration to impact health experiences and outcomes (Spitzer 2016).

Another area of intense research interest, which does account for structural factors, is the concept of incorporation into a host society. Immigrants enter uniquely local "contexts of reception" (Portes & Rumbaut 2001) reflecting the ideology and policies of the receiving location, characteristics and racial makeup of neighborhoods, and conditions of the labor market. These local features fundamentally determine their incorporation trajectories, with implications for the health of individuals and the communities in which they live. Political rhetoric and framing also influence the context of reception that immigrants must navigate to try and adapt to a new social setting (Massey 2020). These narratives may precede or underscore policy decisions and create divisions among groups that establish categories of deservingness – that is, wanted and unwanted categories that ascribe meaning to some immigrants as worthy of compassion while others are viewed only as illegal, at best, or criminals, at worst (Fassin 2011).

Social relationships underlie the health-related effects of integration, including levels of social capital and the accompanying access to resources, both tangible and symbolic (Hacker et al. 2011; Kawachi et al. 2002). Health status is negatively impacted by isolation and economic segregation, which frequently runs along racial or ethnic lines. Immigrants with high levels of social connectedness – for instance those who live in ethnic enclaves or with strong extended kin-based networks – often have strong "bonding" social capital, which can insulate them from effects of discrimination and poverty. "Bridging" social capital can further increase their access to resources such as health care and other services (Kim et al. 2008; Viruell-Fuentes & Schulz 2009). However, access also requires trust in the institutions of a host country, which may be greatly impacted by the presence of police and immigration enforcement activities in communities. Thus, loss of trust further marginalizes already vulnerable populations by reducing bridging social capital (Hacker et al. 2011).

However, the very notion of assimilation rests on static assumptions about intergroup relations and generally posits unidirectional advantages of integration into a host society. In doing so, it often explicitly privileges the position of host societies as desirable or more developed. In recent years, critical race scholars have shifted the focus away from examining immigrant incorporation into receiving societies to instead understanding the ways in which immigrants, their children, and their communities become racialized (Garcia 2017). For migrant communities, this means bringing other axes of stratification – such as undocumented status – into the conversation.

Much of the literature on the association between immigrant assimilation or incorporation relies on crude indicators, such as length of time in the host country, language use, and birthplace as proxy measures of acculturation. This results in weaknesses in explaining health outcomes and a simplistic, linear focus on modifying behavior (Jayaweera 2016). A good example of this is the literature on migration and obesity. Many populations experience weight gain after migrating to host societies where the prevalence of obesity is high (Cairney & Østbye 1999; Sundquist & Johannson 1998; Sundquist & Winkleby 2000). In most cases, studies have noted unhealthy changes in food behaviors after migration, including weight gain, lack of physical activity, and poor diet, including increased consumption of processed food (Himmelgreen et al. 2007). Post-migration lifestyle changes are linked to shifts in pace of life, family interaction, social integration, socioeconomic status, and physical security. Conceptual frameworks frequently presume that migration is the explanation; binational studies suggest that obesity epidemics in both countries of origin and host countries – along with globalization processes that encourage cheap, non-nutritious, highly marketed foods – play a role in poor health outcomes among migrants (Caballero 2007). Yet while some research points to a pattern in which the more acculturated individuals become, the more likely they are to be overweight or obese, other research refutes this (Balcazar et al. 1995; Cairney & Østbye 1999; Khan et al. 1997). This inconsistency is likely due to the imprecise ways in which assimilation or "acculturation" is measured, as well as the degree to which other factors such as education levels and socioeconomic status remain unaccounted for. Therefore, a critical approach is important; a focus on individual dietary behaviors can be misleading and point to the incorrect level for intervention.

Pathogenic Conditions: From Behavioral Explanations to Structural Approaches

Approaches to migrant health have, as we have seen, relied heavily on concepts such as migrant selectivity, health paradoxes, and the effects of acculturation and assimilation (Abraído-Lanza et al. 2005; Acevedo-Garcia & Bates 2007; Antecol & Bedard 2006; Horton & Barker 2010; Hunt et al. 2004). A critical approach must, first, explore the largely unexplored assumptions underlying these, since they generally presume some easily delineated collection of behavioral or "cultural" features, along with the belief that changes in these features are uniform across populations. Shifts over time are viewed as inevitable but rarely as reciprocal. In other words, they leave changes in attitudes and practices of the host country unaddressed, in addition to neglecting variables that impede or accelerate change, such as labor or living conditions. This leads to reductionist approaches that exclude critical structural factors that may be contributing to the deteriorating health of immigrants.

Inequities in the well-being of migrants are heavily determined by factors such as exclusionary policies, discrimination and racism, employment in marginal and dangerous jobs, the high cost of health care, inadequate housing, and poor access to transportation and other resources. Rather than relying on superficial notions of behavioral and cultural change that rest on static assumptions about intergroup relations and unidirectional advantages of assimilation, this book argues instead for understanding the processes of institutional, economic, and political marginalization that continue after they arrive in a new country.

A critical approach begins with the assumption that migration status impacts people's ability to access health-protective resources, as opposed to seeking answers primarily in the loss of "traditional" lifestyle or the behaviors of individuals. These impacts include factors that are external to migrant bodies and are shaped by local and national policies, such as housing conditions, type of employment, and neighborhood safety. For a few of these factors, migrants are explicitly excluded from resources to which other residents are entitled (e.g., preventive care, certain labor protections). For other factors, migrants experience challenges similar to those of other low-income communities, especially communities of color (e.g., racial discrimination, poor housing quality, poor neighborhood safety, food deserts). Undocumented migrants face an additional burden by being unable or unwilling to interact with government services that could provide some relief to their situations; this is out of the (sometimes well-founded) fear that the interaction could lead to arrest, deportation, or family separation.

Thus, in addition to caution regarding behaviorally oriented analyses, it is imperative to move beyond measures of health care access and service utilization and instead look at the ways that political, social, and economic inequalities impose specific risks and constraints on health. These effects may be captured by examining structural factors that are produced by systemic inequalities and social and economic policies (Braveman et al. 2011; Castañeda et al. 2015). This can aid in understanding the effects of conditions such as economic inequalities, structural racism in the housing and employment markets, and gender and ethnic hierarchies, and emphasizes the impact of social structures on the relative positions of individuals and communities in stratified hierarchies and power relationships.

Interactions that lead to socially determined health inequalities are complex and multicausal, requiring investigation of institutional practices and the relationships between macrostructural processes and microlevel behaviors. Among the macrostructural concerns are fundamental social causes of disease (Link & Phelan 1995; Phelan et al. 2010), which can help explain why health inequalities exist under conditions that should eliminate or reduce them, such as advances in medical science or improved access to care. A major focus of this approach is the capacity of individuals and groups to flexibly utilize resources such as knowledge, money, power, prestige, and beneficial social connections; this flexibility (or lack thereof) tells us why and how socioeconomic gradients reproduce themselves over time. Inequalities in health endure primarily because racism is a fundamental cause of disparities in socioeconomic status, and because socioeconomic status is a fundamental cause of health inequalities (Phelan & Link 2015). Finally, notions of "deservingness" can help explain the reasons by which some groups are not considered equally worthy of health-related attention, investment, and care (Holmes 2013; Marrow 2012; Viladrich 2012; Willen 2012). Their inclusion or exclusion is thus linked to larger questions of inequality and the interconnectedness of systems of entitlement.

The range of health challenges associated with migration is wide and often the result of the pathogenic role of social inequality. A syndemics approach understands that these issues exist in interaction, rather than in isolation, and that their epidemiology is a corollary of social context. Indeed, these social conditions "contribute significantly to a biosocial negative feedback loop wherein social and economic inequalities increase the likelihood" of the co-occurrence of diseases (Mendenhall 2016). One example of this, as noted earlier, is diabetes, in which there are frequently co-occurring diseases like hypertension and kidney disease, a syndemic impact of lack of insurance, as well as socio-environmental factors such as income, diet, and lack of transportation. Even though it is complex in its origins, diabetes is often framed as an ethnoracial disease that disproportionately affects Mexican Americans. As a result, research and preventive efforts have a long history of geneticized explanations and presumption of biological difference (Montoya 2007). One effect is the reduction of the disease to a biogenetic condition linked to specific population ancestry or the acculturation level of immigrant groups, and the downplaying of fundamental, lived social conditions in its development and trajectory. Diabetes is a profoundly social condition, for many populations

> brought about by forced migration from rural to urban settings, by an overdetermined reliance on foods with limited nutritional value, by the restrictions of physical movement required of underpaid wage labor and the undercapitalized infrastructure that accompanies it, and by unequal access to health care.
>
> *Montoya 2007: 107–108*

These conditions of poverty, dispossession, and dislocation are fundamental social causes of health inequalities.

Conclusion

Having defined a critical approach and some important terminological considerations, the remainder of the book delves into some specific topical areas associated with migrant health. Even though these areas are highly interconnected and not always easy to parse out into neat categories, each of them offer important theoretical and practical insights. The next chapter examines the migration and transit process specifically along with health-related impacts of border control and immigration policy.

3

HEALTH IN TRANSIT

It was a sweltering Tuesday afternoon in Mazatlán, a coastal city in the state of Sinaloa, Mexico. I sat in a white plastic chair in the dining area of a migrant shelter, listening to a group of young men from El Salvador on their way north. They told stories of violence and the search for a better life; they described having reached their limits in dealing with local gangs in their hometowns, witnessing extortion, rape, even murder. All but one of the men have family members and friends already living in the U.S., who have offered to help them find jobs. These young Salvadorans, like others heading north from Central America, arrived via a freight train often referred to as *la Bestia*, or "the beast." Along the route, they experienced nights unprotected from the cold as the trains traversed mountains, and days in which the sun beat down on them and reinforced already terrible thirst. They faced fistfights with fellow travelers, robbery by local gangs, and intimidation by police in the towns through which they passed.

Later that afternoon, I assisted Dr. Ramirez, a volunteer physician, as he sorted through bags of donated medicines. Most were very near their expiration dates, dropped off by local pharmacies or collected by a local philanthropic organization. As we made piles for different categories – analgesics, topical antibiotics, reflux suppressants, antihistamines, corticosteroids – he described the kinds of complaints he treats at the migrant shelter. Mostly, these are minor injuries like blisters, scrapes and cuts, respiratory illnesses, and gastrointestinal ailments. "Of course," he explained, "These are the lucky ones, the ones that even end up arriving here."

For others, death and dismemberment signal the end of their journey. High-profile stories of mutilations along this transit route are frequent in the media. Shortly after my conversation with the group of Salvadoran men, our research team met Bryan, a 22-year-old from Honduras. He had jumped off *la Bestia* as it pulled into Mazatlán and the heavy train car ran over his left foot, mutilating it severely. Bryan had been in the hospital for three weeks, but the hospital refused to operate

DOI: 10.4324/9781003307532-3

on him until he could pay 35,000 MX pesos (approximately US$1,800 or €1,600). A philanthropic organization sprang into action and collected donations for him, which soon poured in after the community was touched by his story that appeared in the local newspaper. Meanwhile, the hospital's social worker explained that she was required by law to report a migrant patient to immigration authorities; this was part of the protocol, she insisted. As a result of this practice, many migrants leave the hospital without being formally released – and without any follow-up care – to avoid being picked up by authorities.

The stories of the Salvadoran men on their way North and Bryan, stuck in the hospital awaiting surgery, highlight the violence associated with the migrant journey. Over the last decade, transit migration through Mexico has gained importance as several factors continue to drive Central American migration to the U.S. Foremost among them are economic and political insecurity, violence, and underdevelopment. The U.S.' contribution to these "push factors" is well documented – whether through the expansion of "free trade" economic policies or through political support of anti-democratic and quasi-legitimate governments. Current U.S. "aid" to Central America is concentrated primarily on military and police training of the very groups that often contribute to violence against the poor – precisely the violence that drives contemporary outmigration. Policy shifts in the U.S. have further compounded the issue through the mass deportations of migrants accused of criminal offenses, which led to regrouping and strengthening of criminal gangs in Central America. Finally, family-based petitions for legal status remain out of reach for most Central Americans in the U.S., leaving people with few choices other than risking the dangers of clandestine migration.

As the U.S. reinforced security at its southern border, it put pressure on its neighbor Mexico to increase interior enforcement by setting up checkpoints along major highways, expanding detention facilities, and stepping up deportations through agreements with Central American countries. The U.S. has given Mexico hundreds of millions of dollars to stop migrants from reaching its border to claim asylum, essentially "outsourcing" the problem to Mexico through programs such as Plan Frontera Sur (2014) and Migrant Protection Protocols (2019, also called the "Remain in Mexico" program). Meanwhile, transit through Mexico had become more hazardous as migrants have been subject to frequent victimization; the highly publicized incident occurred in August 2010, when 72 migrants were found dead in Tamaulipas at the hands of the Zetas, a criminal organization known to extort migrants passing through their territories. This is in addition to the already treacherous conditions; a majority of migrant border deaths are related to heat exposure (in 2021, at least 650 people died attempting to cross the U.S.-Mexico border; IOM 2022); others have died due to suffocation in tractor-trailers along the way.

This chapter provides an overview of the health-related impacts of border control policies and practices. It explores the dynamics that shape migratory flows and the risks and vulnerabilities of unauthorized (or irregular) movements. It frames impacts on health as located within the rise in the militarization of borders across the globe and a fundamental dilemma between ongoing demand for migrant labor and the lack of opportunities to cross borders legally. When people are compelled to enact mobility in unauthorized manner, it results in specific and often violent risks to health, including death. Taking transit itself as a site of theoretical inquiry, it seeks to move the discussion beyond the binaries of push/pull factors and origin/destination countries, with analytical implications for understanding vulnerability, risk, and inequality, as well as encounters of care. Forced immobility is a common pattern around the globe today, and so health is impacted not only by border crossings themselves but also during time spent waiting in border zones, refugee camps, migrant shelters, and detention centers. Related to this, borders themselves now frequently transcend physical space and reach into spaces of everyday life as strategic sites subject to intensified policing. Finally, this chapter examines the health impacts of family separation through migration, as well as the positive and negative impacts of cross-border ties. The key questions that this chapter answers include, How does the precarity of migrants' journeys affect risk and vulnerability? How is "illegality" produced through bordering practices and intensified policing, and what are the implications on health? How is well-being impacted by family separation? How is it impacted by maintaining ties to country of origin?

Critical Approaches to Understanding Health in Transit

To understand illness and injury associated with mobilities and specifically while in transit, we must understand the role of larger political, economic, and securitization efforts and how they constrain and facilitate certain patterns. A critical approach emphasizes the deeper historical and political roots of particular migrations to avoid reductionist and merely technical approaches to understanding migrant injury and illness. Returning to the introductory vignette of the chapter, this means that the larger sociopolitical context of Bryan's case is just as important as the medical treatment plan that the physicians and nurses tried to devise for him, given their own constraints. The wheel that almost severed his leg was attached to a beast of a freight train that had already taken countless other lives and limbs. This train is a vehicle of both hope and terror for thousands heading north, illuminating the underlying conditions that compel people to migrate steeped in decades of imperialism, extractionist policies, and border militarization. Training the lens on specific interactions in the Mexican hospital means being attuned to local and regional dynamics with implications for encounters of care and solidarity (e.g., donations by the local community) as well as interior border enforcement (e.g., policies that compel medical staff to report Bryan to immigration authorities). Every day around the globe, medical dilemmas result from these complex inequalities, as migration is the result of broader political and economic processes that displace populations.

This chapter provides an overview of the health-related impacts of border control and immigration policy. Using the principles laid out in Chapter 2, it takes a critical approach by explicitly attending to the exercise and distribution of power.

It problematizes the concept of "the border" as a naturalized object, instead framing it as highly malleable and contingent. While this chapter focuses on the journey, it also recognizes that migration is not easily split into discrete "phases," and the epistemic divide between "country of origin" and "destination" is often ambiguous. The binary positioning of sending country/host country has become increasingly blurred. Transit migration occurs as people stop in places between origin and intended destination, sometimes for short periods of time and sometimes for many years. During this period, migrants may experience significant health risks, physical danger, exposure to violence, trauma, hunger and thirst, and poor access to medical care even in emergency situations. Finally, as this chapter emphasizes, the journey does not end with "arrival" to a "host" country; rather, migration is a process that takes many directions with implications for conventional notions of space and time, as well as for the well-being of communities for generations to come.

Violence of Border Controls and Production of Illegality

Since the 1990s, there has been a rise in the militarization of borders worldwide. Especially since the early 2000s, migration has been portrayed as a security threat to be constantly monitored, with protectionist policies producing adverse consequences on the very lives of migrants (Andersson 2014a; De León 2015; Thomas 2016). As the opening to this chapter described, in the U.S. a set of policies have been instituted with the intent to deter the illegal crossing of its southern border with Mexico. A set of policies in the 1990s referred to as "Prevention through Deterrence" created a funnel effect through the most dangerous parts of the Sonoran desert, resulting in a shocking number of migrant deaths (De León 2015). Rather than deterring unauthorized migration, these policies have had the effect of increasing smuggling operations and mortality rates of those crossing the border (Nevins 2001), using the natural hazards and geographic space of the desert as a "moral alibi" (Doty 2011) to avoid official responsibility for migrant deaths. Today, this weaponization of the natural environment has been complemented with the erection of portions of a wall, fencing, drones, blimps, underground sensors, and increased presence of Border Patrol agents.

Meanwhile, in Europe, increasingly restrictive national policies since the 1990s and the militarization of the outer boundary of the EU have created what has become known as "Fortress Europe." Attempts to cross into Europe via the Mediterranean have become increasingly deadly (Andersson 2014a), with migrant deaths at sea playing an instrumental role in shaping policy and public responses. However, these "geographies of violence and death" stretch throughout the migration process and begin far away from the Mediterranean shores (McMahon & Sigona 2021). People's exposure to death is a fundamental part of trajectories stretching across many months and thousands of kilometers, shaping not only the decision to migrate but also the evolution of their journeys. Indeed, these experiences frequently have cumulative implications for how people interpret risks and make decisions along the way (McMahon & Sigona 2021).

Other nations have implemented even more deadly border control practices. India, for example, has adopted shoot-to-kill practices since 2002 against Bangladeshi immigrants crossing the border, resulting in the deaths of thousands (Oztig 2016). Rather than utilizing walls, fencing, and surveillance through technology, it has relied on shooting practices associated with arbitrariness; policymakers from a wide policy spectrum have legitimized any method to curb illegal immigration, and the Indian legal system allows agents of the Border Security Force impunity to carry out these activities (Oztig 2016).

Unauthorized and often clandestine border crossings create specific risks to health, increasing bodily trauma, hunger, and thirst, as well as dangerous exposures to interpersonal violence and the physical environment (crossing large bodies of water, mountains, or inhospitable deserts). This is coupled with little to no access to medical care. Violence affects some groups more than others; it is often highly gendered, with women particularly vulnerable to sexual assault as part of the systematic degradation that accompanies militarization practices (Green 2011). Children separated from their families during migration are highly vulnerable to violence (Mason-Jones & Nicholson 2018), especialy dangerous for those fleeing conflict and persecution (Digidiki & Bhabha 2017; Human Rights Watch 2016; UNICEF 2017). Children are also often the most vulnerable to exploitation and abuse during transit due to exposure to traffickers, loss of social and familial structures, and physical and emotional immaturity (Morof et al. 2014; Thornton & Veenema 2015).

Around the globe, these "border spectacles" highlight what appear to be contradictory processes: an ongoing need for and tolerance of undocumented labor, coupled with a lack of opportunities to cross borders legally. One major strategy of deterrence is constructing unauthorized migrants as criminals who threaten the safety of citizens. This rhetoric rests on a logic situating the migrant outside the protection of the legal system, essentially as a "non-person" to whom the state has no obligation (Inda & Dowling 2013). This framing of illegality (and of human beings as "illegals" who have violated the law) permits and encourages violent responses, including persecution, detention, and deportation. This has the effect of racializing and illegalizing particular groups, such as sub-Saharan Africans in Europe and Latin Americans (and especially Mexicans) in the U.S. Migrants' vulnerability when illegally crossing borders must be situated within a complex web of capitalist relations that produce at an unprecedented rate a shared experience of "disposable people who have been displaced and dislocated from their means of survival" (Green 2011: 366). The state's capacity to decide who will be disproportionately exposed to death – as one expression of the operation of sovereignty – has been referred to as *necroviolence* (Mbembé 2003), especially evident in border control practices described here. A critical perspective locates these deaths squarely in structural conditions of inequality, rather than the choices of individuals to migrate.

Forced Immobility and Stuckness

Critical studies of migration have expanded beyond the limits of "origin" and "destination" to analytically map zones of transit as imperative sites of investigation in contemporary global migration flows. In doing so, transit migration is revealed to be comprised of encounters that push us to reconsider the social and physical spaces of migrant journeys and the impacts of these encounters not only for the migrants themselves but for state and non-state actors of local communities through which they pass. Thus, the idea of "transit" migration or "transit" countries can effectively challenge the traditional dichotomy of mobility and immobility, or of sending and receiving countries.

There has been increased interest in the phenomenon of "transit" and people's intermittent stays at the fringes of Europe, the U.S., and other migrant destinations (Andersson 2014a; Basok et al. 2015; Düvell 2006; Mainwaring & Brigden 2016; Phillips & Missbach 2017; Schapendonk 2012; Vogt 2018). One productive way to think about this is by distinguishing between journeys and transit experiences; the former is (generally) shorter and (maybe) unidirectional, whereas the latter may represent extended periods of time in unintended places. Yet the concept of "transit migration" has been problematized in recent years for implying an empty in-betweenness, wandering about, or a waiting process. It most often refers to a kind of "ongoing mobility" (Düvell 2006) or to a period of involuntary immobility (Schapendonk 2007, 2012, 2013), in which people become "stuck" in a place (Carling 2007; Missbach 2015; Stock 2019). There are several contexts of migrant immobilization, such as border zones (Castañeda & Melo 2019); Mainwaring & Brigden 2016), refugee camps (Malkki 1996; Redclift 2013b), migrant shelters (Balaguera 2018, 2019), and detention centers (Fassin 2005), all of which have the potential to produce immobilization, new social realities (Andersson 2014a; Basok et al. 2015), and new forms of care and solidarity (Vogt 2018).

Indeed, migrant "stuckness" and the condition of waiting is a growing pattern around the globe today (Alioua 2017; Andersson 2014a; Bachelet 2019; Basok et al. 2015; Düvell 2006; Jacobsen et al. 2021; Phillips & Missbach 2017; Schapendonk 2012; Stock 2019; Vogt 2018). There is a move toward defining transit migration from the perspective of migrants' precarity rather than the mostly Euro-centric policy-driven definitions, which tend to view Western countries as the only, primary, or preferred destinations in the migrant imagination. Particularly in the European context,

> the term 'transit country' generally refers to the countries on the fringes of the EU, accentuating further the presumption of the exteriority of these countries and the idea that a 'natural' border separates the EU from the rest of the world.
>
> *Alioua 2017: 152*

Several alternative frameworks have been developed, such as "fragmented journeys" (Collyer 2007, 2010), in which migrants are forced to wait for indefinite periods until new opportunities arise, as well as a focus on the rich and complex social relationships forged in "transit" sites and temporalities (Bachelet 2019).

These understandings of transit zones allow us to account for the experiences of increasing numbers of migrants "stuck in mobility," with all its complexity, unsteadiness, and multidirectionality. Waiting and the temporalities of irregular migration take on novel forms (Jacobsen et al. 2021; Khosravi 2010), as people are not only subjected to extended periods of waiting but also face active usurpation or appropriation of their time by state authorities through serial expulsions and detention practices (Andersson 2014b). In transit contexts, people's health is impacted by the harms they face not only during border crossings but also during time spent working, living, and waiting along the way.

Smuggling and Trafficking

A brief examination of the concepts "trafficking" and "smuggling" are in order when discussing migration, as these are often used interchangeably in the media and in policy discussions. In practice, the distinction between them is not always a clear one, despite very different notions of agency and intent. Smuggling describes the crossing of international borders, in which consenting individuals are assisted (although the concept of consent can be problematized, since they may not have full agency), whereas legal definitions of trafficking focus on situations of fraud, force, or coercion, in which actual movement is not a required component. Put another way, while trafficking may be part of the migration experience, migration is not a required part of the trafficking experience. Some scholars have focused on these characteristics of the "customer relationship" to determine whether a situation is considered trafficking and smuggling (Iselin & Adams 2003). In smuggling, the "customer" is essentially the one being smuggled, whereas in trafficking, the customer is the purchaser of a "commodity" (i.e., a trafficked person). In other words, in distinguishing these practices, what matters is the level of agency – or, conversely, the lack thereof in the form of coercion.

The overrepresentation of trafficking in migration scholarship is misleading, especially because of the disproportionate focus on sex trafficking. Anti-trafficking discourses perpetuated by NGOs and the media consistently conflate sex work and trafficking, relying on the trope of the "iconic victim" (Srikantiah 2007), especially innocent women. Cultural oppression, including racism and ethnic bias, creates additional and often overlooked risks for trafficking, generating unique challenges for prevention and intervention (Bryant-Davis & Tummala-Narra 2017). On the whole, the difficulty of recognizing and establishing more precise definitions of "victims of trafficking" impacts health care for this population, especially evident in policy gaps in the provision of social and medical services. The overemphasis on sex trafficking also obscures from public and policy view the large number of labor trafficking violations, which are picked up and discussed again in Chapter 7.

A focus on smuggling practices and relationships is thus more appropriately tied to migration processes, especially as they relate to experiences in transit.

However, research in this area suffers from conceptual "messiness" and competing understandings and norms about how to interpret migrant smuggling (Baird & van Liempt 2016). As it is used in the media, as well as in popular discourse and policy circles, the term is heavily dominated by policing perspectives. Critical scholars, on the other hand, have pointed to the fact that – contrary to the popular image of smugglers as dangerous criminals – smugglers are often migrants themselves, who facilitate illegal journeys, entry, and/or legalization of family members, friends, or strangers who pay them a fee.

The smuggling business is thus a socially embedded phenomenon, carrying with it more positive and pragmatic associations among migrants than from the point of view of outsiders. While in transit, migrants frequently become embedded in local and transnational economies of smuggling, and a close examination of these experiences can contribute to reconceptualizing human smuggling as a form of *intimate labor* along migrant routes (Vogt 2016). In contrast to conventional understandings of smuggling as inherently exploitative, these transactions can be seen as a point of intimate exchange as people strategically reimagine the borders of kinship. In this light, the social relations forged in transit between migrants and their smugglers illuminate larger arrangements of inequality.

Respatialization of Border Controls: Externalization and Internalization Practices

In addition to reconfigured spaces between origins and destinations, borders are no longer simply physical delineations that mark out the edge of a state, regulating movement across them. Beginning in the 1990s and intensifying in the decades since, borders have been increasingly pushed to the *interior* of nation-states and are becoming disaggregated to reach into spaces of everyday life as strategic sites now subject to intensified policing. Today, borders have become a "mobile technology – a portable, diffused, and decentered control apparatus interwoven throughout the nation" (Dowling & Inda 2013: 145). Work by critical security scholars has emphasized the respatialization of borders and the ways in which technologies – biometric identity systems, digital surveillance, and databanking – have produced networked, contingent borders that transcend physical boundaries and appear to be both everywhere and nowhere at the same time (Coleman 2012; Rosas 2006).

Today, securitization practices and discourse dominate migration management, with increased reliance on border enforcement, detention, and deportation as strategies to control unauthorized movements. Across the globe a similar trend emerged, particularly after the September 11, 2001, attacks, moving policy and practice ever further away from international humanitarian guidelines. That was a pivotal moment in which security concerns became the key driver of immigration policy in many countries (Dickson 2015), leading to increased militarization and fortification of borders. Inspection and policing practices have expanded both within and beyond territorial boundaries, as contemporary securitization-oriented migration management relies on dual processes of externalization (i.e., outsourcing activities to sending and transit countries as an extension of legal regimes) and internalization of border controls (Menjívar 2014). This has expanded migration management both beyond the physical international border and toward the interior of states, accompanied by the proliferation of inspection checkpoints, surveillance technologies, and detention practices. This is most visibly the case in the EU and the U.S., as they encountered the two greatest refugee movements to unfold in this century.

Externalization refers to the "offshoring" or outsourcing of activities to sending and transit countries as an extension of border control and its associated legal regimes. To return to the North American example, the U.S. has increasingly utilized its neighbor Mexico as a buffer zone for those trying to immigrate north, funneling money, technology, and training to assist Mexico in fortifying its southern border. Migration policies in Mexico have also become increasingly restrictive, especially following 2018, when thousands of Central Americans traveled through Mexico in caravans toward the U.S. border. This humanitarian crisis compelled Mexico to further enact restrictive securitization measures in response to both internal and external (U.S.) political pressures. Meanwhile, on the U.S. side, a program called the Migrant Protection Protocols (also known as the "Remain in Mexico" program) was initiated in 2019 that enabled the U.S. to send non-Mexican asylum seekers back to Mexico to await immigration proceedings. It was an unprecedented extension of prior externalization efforts, since it introduced a new "safe third country" rule that has variably been viewed as unlawful and reversing the country's legal and moral commitment to protect those fleeing danger. The program was temporarily suspended in response to the COVID-19 pandemic, leaving over 14,000 asylum seekers trapped in northern Mexico without adequate resources including housing and sanitation.

In the EU, migration control has relied on the "off-shoring" and "out-sourcing" of borders as a primary strategy for decades. Unlike the North American case, the EU operates through a more fluid assemblage of processes, institutional arrangements, and actors, recomposing spaces as necessary (Bialasiewicz 2012). For example, FRONTEX, created in 2005, which promotes, organizes, and develops European border management, is formally constituted as simply a "regulatory agency" responsible for coordination between member states on issues related to border control. However, it is undoubtedly the de facto border patrol and most visible actor in the EU's exclusionary bordering practices.

Externalization processes in the EU operate through funding, training, and cooperation agreements with the entire Mediterranean region along with neighboring countries such as Ukraine, Belarus, and Moldova. As one critical migration scholar notes "EUrope's neighbours are, in other words, becoming EUrope's policemen" (Bialasiewicz 2012: 847). The securitization of Mediterranean by the EU has pushed bordering processes to north Africa, especially Libya, Morocco, Algeria, and Mauritania. This has resulted in hundreds of thousands of deportations and "return migrants" to Africa; many of these return operations have been implemented from so-called "transit countries," thus pushing the boundaries of the EU well into another continent.

Critical border studies have been particularly attentive to the local effects of Europe's externalization of border control, especially as it has attempted to move toward a "softer" and "more humanist" approach to managing migration. These efforts have had the effect of producing new, contested border zones with the goal of further obstructing mobility. EU-driven migration management regimes have been critiqued for their disconnection from local politics and mobility practices in countries of origin, transit, and reception (Sylla & Cold-Ravnkilde 2021), spurring much discontent and contestation. Narratives of voluntary return also obscure how repatriation happens in the context of human rights violations, including unlawful deportations and inhumane detention in, for example, Libya (Alpes 2020). These externalization processes end up pushing responsibility for migrants in distress onto their poorer neighbors, with wealthy destination countries denying people access to vital humanitarian protection on their territory in contravention of binding legal obligations (Digidiki & Bhabha 2021). By putting into place such deliberate policies and practices to deter migration, these countries also knowingly and willfully relegate distress migrants to areas known for rampant violence, which is especially concerning given the rapidly growing number of vulnerable people, such as children (Digidiki & Bhabha 2021).

In another case of externalization, Australia has, since 2001, had a mandatory immigration detention system for "unlawful non-citizens" that includes offshore locations on the Pacific island of Nauru and Manus Island in Papua New Guinea. It thus follows a pre-emptive strategy to curb illegal entry through increased maritime policy instruments and unique practices of detention and repatriation for irregular migrants intercepted at sea (Dickson 2015). The Australian government has funded privately operated offshore immigration detention centers, in which asylum seekers are detained, mandatorily and indefinitely, while they wait on the processing of their claims. This practice has drawn a great deal of attention as it combines remote locations and prolonged poor detention conditions, which have been shown to severely impact asylum seekers' physical and mental health (Hedrick et al. 2020), specifically in relation to self-harm.

Internalized border controls often accompany such externalization practices. In many places, the physical border has quite literally moved to the interior, with checkpoints operating to further control movement. In the southwest U.S., for example, a series of permanent checkpoints creates a sense of regional confinement that affects the lives of all immigrants, regardless of whether they are recent arrivals or have lived in the U.S. for decades (Castañeda & Melo 2019). These checkpoints are located between 25 and 100 miles from the border along all major highways that lead into the interior of the U.S. and are staffed 24 hours a day, seven days a week, forcing all travelers to pass through them. These permanent checkpoints are supplemented by unpredictable temporary roadblocks placed in communities where immigrants live and work, operating as an additional level of inspection, creating an environment of entrapment, and resulting in what some have referred to as a state of carcelment (Dorsey & Díaz-Barriga 2015). Indeed, spatial containment and immobility are part of the logics of border control, in this case by creating additional borders beyond the international boundary. The containment of immigrants in places like along the U.S./Mexico border is an example of the complex spatial implications of the securitization of migration management (Coutin 2010) as it produces marginalized spaces with particular consequences for the people who inhabit them.

Finally, another layer of bordering practices occur via unpredictable and unsettling raids, detentions, and deportations. One result of the uncertainty associated with these forms of policing is the avoidance of interactions with the state and its authorities, including in the form of medical attention. A major impact of the respatialization of borders via checkpoints, raids, detentions, and deportations is the separation of families, which is discussed in further detail in Chapter 10. These "spectacular forms of violence" (Goldstein 2010, see also De Genova 2013) are rituals that aim to deter further migration by creating an environment of insecurity and vulnerability (of immigrants) in the name of security (of citizens). As arbitrary public expressions of state power, they function to instruct by destabilizing communities through the criminalization of non-citizens.

Family Shifts and Separation through Migration

Also related to health in transit are the familial separations and transnational connections that accompany the migration process. As global inequalities drive people to seek work elsewhere to provide for their children, migration is a key driver of fundamental shifts in household structure and family composition. Scholarship in this area has noted the effects of migration on changes in marriage and conjugal relations, transnational parenting practices, and the reconfiguring of family structures (Wurtz & Castañeda forthcoming).

Family separations, especially between parents and children, are particularly frequent during migration, though the duration of this separation varies widely. Parents may choose or have no option but to leave their children for a variety of reasons: journeys maybe too dangerous to travel as a family unit, immigration policies may not permit family unification, or jobs may be too precarious with long hours, making it difficult to simultanously care for children. Historically, the more common pattern has been males migrating by themselves, although sometimes the parental couple will migrate together or it is the mother who leaves the children behind. However, mothers' migrations tend to be the most reluctant, as research in a number of settings has illustrated (Ehrenreich et al. 2003; Hondagneu-Sotelo 2001; Parrenas 2001). Most often the decision is taken out of economic neccessity, in cases where jobs may be more lucrative for women (e.g., in carework with children, the elderly, or in medical settings). Not infrequently, children are left to live with their grandparents; this intergenerational care often reconfigures relationships in communities as it serves as a resource for the well-being of children and other family members who stay behind (Yarris 2017).

Family separation, ultimately due to policies that restrict migration opportunities, may create emotional hardships for children, with many reporting emotional distress and resentment (Coe 2021; Coe et al. 2011; Dreby 2010). Their performance in school may suffer when compared with children who do not experience separation (Jensen et al. 2016; McKenzie & Rapoport 2006). Prolonged family separation has been shown to serve as a risk factor for mental health and overall well-being (Menjívar & Abrego 2012). This goes for the parents as well; in a study of Latina immigrants in the U.S., rates of depression were found to be significantly higher among women who left behind children in countries of origin, when compared to those who were still living with their children (Menjívar & Abrego 2012).

At the same time, not all separation via parental migration is extraordinary, probematic, or harmful. There are a number of social contexts in which migration has a long history well-embedded in community and family life, with separation one part of a calculus that includes material benefits and representations of love by parents toward their children (Chamberlain 2006; Olwig 1999; Poeze & Mazzucato 2013). Indeed, migration-related separation from family and friends has been found to have both adverse and beneficial outcomes, often moderated by the strength of cross-border ties (Torres 2013).

Cross-Border Ties: Implications for Health

Despite crossing borders, many migrants still maintain strong ties to their host country. Migration frequently separates spouses, parents and children, and extended family members, in addition to affecting the closeness of friendships and people's other affective connections to their home communities. However, social, economic, religious, and other ties are maintained through return travel, seasonal pendular movements, frequent calls and messages, remittances, active participation in politics while abroad, involvement in compatriot or coethnic associations, and maintaining businesses and property in home communities. Remittances have sharply increased in recent decades, from \$126 billion in 2000 to \$702 billion in 2020 (IOM 2022); even during the pandemic, there was only a slight drop (2.4%) in the global total, despite predictions of a large decline. These ongoing ties illustrate that there is frequently no clear epistemic distinction between "here" and "there," and that the social lives of migrants are not tethered to the host country but rather are influenced by home communities as well.

But how do these cross-border connections impact health? Research on the connections between transnational/binational communities sheds light on both negative and positive associations – that is, not only in the potential risks that are "carried" but also in practices of resilience. A growing number of studies, most focused on Latino immigrants in the U.S. (Alcántara et al. 2015a, 2015b; Torres 2013), have found significant associations between cross-border social ties and immigrant health outcomes. Most have focused on mental health, health behaviors, and self-rated subjective well-being; nonetheless, there is evidence that these have direct physical health outcomes on, for example, cardiovascular disease and other chronic health conditions (Yang et al. 2016).

On the one hand, cross-border ties appear to be protective for mental health and subjective well-being by facilitating continued cohesion with family and community, despite the separation caused by migration. This helps uphold a sense of belonging and purpose, and family members back home may provide important emotional support for migrants living abroad, especially if they are experiencing social isolation (Viruell-Fuentes & Schulz 2009). Cross-border ties may serve as a source of information about health conditions and other concerns. Continued familiar dietary practices and the delivery of "care packages" help migrants to uphold ties to their communities (Handley et al. 2013). In addition, economic ties in the form of remittances can elevate migrants' social standing and levels of prestige in their home communities, in addition to providing financially for their family. This may contribute to positive health outcomes through upward socioeconomic mobility and a sense of fulfilling one's obligations (Alcántara et al. 2015a; Carling 2014). However, as one study of Arab Americans concluded, the relationship between cross-border ties and psychological distress and happiness was complex and varied by generation (Samari 2016).

On the other hand, there are numerous ways in which cross-border ties may negatively impact well-being. As noted above, family separation affects mental health, with even greater adverse impacts for those lacking sufficient financial resources or ability (especially because of their undocumented or irregular status) to make return visits to their countries of origin. Furthermore, people may experience stress due to the multiple social and economic obligations and expectations, creating both financial strain and social burden. This distress may be amplified if they occupy marginal social positions in host countries, where they face poverty, unfulfilling or dangerous jobs, and discrimination. On a physical level, prolonged stress related to cross-border family separation may contribute to greater systemic inflammation (Torres et al. 2018), as well as coping behaviors that have negative consequences for health (e.g., smoking).

These effects are often highly gendered; for instance, male migrants frequently face greater social expectations to provide remittances despite low wages; for women, caring for children may add additional pressures that negatively impact health. Transnational motherhood (Hondagneu-Sotelo & Avila 1997) refers to situations in which women must negotiate caregiving while separated from their children, as they try to maintain mothering ties through financial remittances, frequent phone calls, and photos. In addition, other forms of transnational caregiving – especially for elderly family members – increases the burden on women, in particular (Viruell-Fuentes 2006). Research on transnational activities in several very different contexts confirms these highly gendered differences, as women disproportionately provide emotional and logistic support to family in their countries of origin, including children, aging parents, and siblings (Abrego 2014; Fouron & Schiller 2001; Viruell-Fuentes 2006). There are also uniquely gendered obligations to send home remittances, as one study on Ghanaian transnational families highlighted, despite women's disproportionately precarious status and work conditions (Wong 2006). A study on the health of sub-Saharan African migrants living in France found that remitting money and being separated from children were each associated with poor health among women, but not men. This underscores the importance of examining differential impacts by gender in the study of cross-border connections in migrant health (Afulani et al. 2016).

Conclusion

This chapter has examined how the precarity of migrants' journeys impacts risk and vulnerability, locating this precarity in processes of illegality and the militarization of borders worldwide. Locating these "border spectacles," it highlighted what appear to be contradictory processes: a need for undocumented labor coupled with a lack of opportunities to cross borders legally. Importantly, not all migrants cross borders clandestinely or without authorization. In many cases – one might even say in most cases, depending on the country – undocumented or irregular status is the result of overstaying the duration of a (e.g., tourist or student) visa, rather than illegal entry, a fact that is often overshadowed by the border spectacles highlighted in the media and in policy debates. Unauthorized and often clandestine forms of border crossings create specific risks to health, even as borders themselves have been respatialized and frequently transcend physical space to reach into everyday life. One major strategy of deterrence, as we have seen, is constructing unauthorized migrants as criminals who threaten the safety of citizens. "Illegality" is produced and reinforced through securitization practices and discourse that now dominate migration management, and which include externalization and internalization bordering practices. Finally, this chapter examined how well-being is impacted by family separation, with disproportionate impacts on women worldwide, and how maintaining ties to country of origin can have both positive and negative effects on health.

The next chapter examines experiences on arrival to a host country to interrogate the policy-level influences on immigrant and refugee health. Depending on the specific setting, migrants are more or less excluded from formal systems of health care, often due to differential constructions and discourses of "deservingness," which deem them unwanted, undesirable, and undeserving of resources and ensuring continued marginalization. This chapter examines access to and utilization of health care, including the web of barriers migrants face in host countries and the ways in which the politics of care create new forms of inequality.

4

HEALTH CARE ACCESS AND UTILIZATION

Veronica is a 38-year-old mother of five children – three born in the U.S. and two in Mexico. She and her husband, who are both undocumented, along with the two older children, came to the U.S. eight years before I spoke with her in her home in South Texas. They were a typical mixed-status family, juggling the various restrictions and opportunities for each family member because of their varied legal status. Veronica described the odyssey that ensued when her children get sick:

> Well, for the citizen children who have Medicaid, I call their pediatrician. If they are very sick, they will even be seen the same day. But for the older two, I have to take them to El Milagro [a local charity clinic]. They are only open certain days and certain hours and there is always a long line. And I don't have a car, so if my husband is working, then I have to ask a neighbor to take us. It's a lot of stress!

Different legal statuses result in divergent opportunities when it comes to medical care in mixed-status immigrant families. Parents like Veronica must cultivate the ability to take care of some health care needs at home in addition to seeking services in multiple sites with distinct plans for individual members depending on their status. U.S.-born children with Medicaid – a medical benefits program that provides public assistance to low-income persons who qualify – can visit private physician practices, while undocumented and/or uninsured individuals must avoid getting sick. When siblings with different forms of health care access became ill at the same time, as is often the case with colds and other common childhood infections, mothers like Veronica spent the greater part of a day or more first visiting a pediatrician, followed by long waits at a charity clinic or community health center hoping to have an undocumented child seen for the same condition. This results in time off from work and loss of income. As Veronica pointed out, this can be

DOI: 10.4324/9781003307532-4

logistically difficult if no transportation is available, and there are no buses or taxis that serve the rural neighborhood in which she lives.

Later I spoke with Javier, Veronica's 18-year-old son. He was brought to the U.S. at the age of ten alongside his younger sister, while his three younger brothers were all born in Texas. Growing up, he and his sister were undocumented like their parents. Javier considered his brothers to be "lucky" by virtue of their place of birth, which affords them access to treatment in times of acute illness, regular checkups, and dental care. The rest of the family must go without these benefits. Like many other undocumented children in mixed-status families, he recalled that his parents often told him to "not get sick." He said, "I remember if we would get sick, and it was like, 'Suck it up. We don't have money to take you to a doctor.' There wasn't much we could do" (Castañeda 2019).

Eligibility for health care coverage in the U.S. is significantly determined by legal status. While U.S. citizens under the age of 18 can access Medicaid and the Children's Health Insurance Program, undocumented children and parents are ineligible for all publicly funded services besides perinatal and emergency medical care. Even if they were, these do not necessarily provide a guarantee of comprehensive access. Given the low income levels for immigrant families, most are not able to private pay for medical services out of pocket.

Based on this example from the U.S., the experiences of Veronica's family illustrate how immigration policies and health care intersect at numerous junctures. These policies have multiple direct and indirect impacts specifically on these families, including their hesitancy to enroll citizen children in programs due to fear of deportation or to avoid jeopardizing chances of future regularization. There is little doubt that the rise in anti-immigrant policymaking has fostered an unhealthy environment for immigrants and their families. They report worse physical health compared to their citizen counterparts, and hostile immigration policies further exacerbate these health disparities.

This chapter begins by exploring the policy-level influences on migrants' access to health, examining how laws in the receiving country impact differential treatment and outcomes. Using a comparative approach, it examines the policy environment in various host nations, illustrating that migrants are generally excluded from systems of health care promotion and provision (Falge & Ruzza 2016). These policies create differential constructions of migrants seeking health care (Alunni 2015; Horton 2004) and produce discourses of "deservingness," which deem them unwanted, undesirable, and undeserving of protection or public support, thus ensuring their continued marginalization (Willen 2012). The coupling of securitization and humanitarianism (Ticktin 2011) can further compromise well-being. Even in purportedly universal health care systems, migrants are systematically excluded due to bureaucratic disentitlement and requirements to report their presence to the authorities. There is a disconnect between obligations under international rights conventions and how access to health care is translated in daily practice. As charities and humanitarian organizations step in to provide necessary services, they sometimes legitimize shrinking public safety nets by complicating discourses about entitlement, further stratifying populations. Yet the health-related inequalities resulting from exclusion motivate people to organize on migrants' behalf, frequently based on local configurations of legitimacy (Willen et al. 2011). These ambivalent policies have resulted in two-tiered medical systems in many host countries as well as a proliferation of services performed by NGOs and charity clinics. Rather than anchored in policy or rights, these efforts offer only short-term, improvisational remedies, often in the name of sympathy and generosity. The key questions that this chapter answers include the following: How do policies impact migrants' access to health care? What are the health service utilization patterns for migrants? How do migrants fare in "universal" health care systems? What is the impact of NGOs that step in to provide care?

Critical Approaches to Understanding Health Care Access and Utilization

Migrants' patterned lack of access to health care services constitutes a burgeoning global health challenge. Yet one of the key contradictions is that even though access to medical care is frequently restricted for them out of concern that they will drain resources, migrants actually use fewer services than their citizen counterparts, in addition to often having a more robust health profile, as mentioned in Chapter 2. And while many do have health insurance and utilize services, these are often not available at the same level or at the same quality as for citizens. Without sufficient inclusion to the health care system, migrants (especially undocumented migrants) face limited diagnosis and treatment, so that major health issues remain unaddressed until they are an emergency. They are also frequently forced to accept higher occupational health risks compared to citizens; as a result, they become trapped in systems of precarity, which, in turn, foster additional exclusions. A critical approach to access issues recognizes how these exclusions serve larger frameworks of power, nativist ideologies, and neoliberal economic systems.

There is also a vast disconnect between obligations under international conventions and how health care policy is translated in daily practice. Universal notions of a "right to health" often operate together with incongruous local, state, national, and international policies, all with different ethicolegal grounds for entitlements. A critical approach that starts with the political and historical framing context can uncover patterns in constructions of deservingness and in the web of barriers migrant populations face in accessing care (Čebron 2010; Falge & Ruzza 2016; Goldade 2009; Gottlieb et al. 2012; Rosenthal 2007; Willen 2012). Migrant "illegality" is simultaneously a juridical status and a sociopolitical condition (De Genova 2002), and processes of "illegalization" challenge us to consider health-related deservingness, or the moral ways in which some groups, but not others, are considered deserving of attention, investment, and care (Willen 2012). Because they interact with poor living and labor conditions to foster increased susceptibility to ill health, these "pathologizing politics of alienhood" are literally marked on migrant bodies (Marciniak 2006: xiii).

Policy Frameworks Determining Access to Medical Care

Access to medical care is the primary structural factor affecting migrant health. Although policies that regulate health care vary greatly in terms of times, place, and specificity, overall, migrants (especially undocumented migrants) experience limited access, which is often a downstream product of larger structural or colonial conditions, requiring a critical approach to analyzing both social and policy determinants. Access to health care may also be strongly linked to ethno-national conceptions of citizenship, as has been argued in the case of Israel, among other examples (Filc & Davidovich 2005).

There are numerous misconceptions regarding unauthorized migration and health care. As noted earlier, empirical evidence has repeatedly shown that undocumented migrants use fewer services than legal residents (Wolff et al. 2008) and that migration occurs in response to economic conditions, not to gain access to social services. Furthermore, in most instances, migrants have lower rates of health care use, and their health tends to deteriorate the longer they reside in the host country (Berk et al. 2000; Chacón & Davis 2006). Excluding unauthorized migrants from receiving publicly funded medical services and programs is unlikely to have an impact of immigration patterns, as evidenced over and over, and in fact may have negative effects on citizens, such as migrants' children born in the host country.

Migration policy is often intimately intertwined with health care policy, and frequently subject to polemical debate. Efforts aimed at deterring migration often manifest themselves as restrictions on public benefits and social services to migrants, especially by limiting health care options (Berk et al. 2000; Fassin 2005; Düvell & Jordan 2002). In the U.S., for instance, policies on migrant health have always been contradictory, fragmentary, or non-existent, although over the past three decades, the legal climate has become increasingly hostile (Hoffman 2006). Several proposals restricting and even criminalizing medical assistance have circulated. California's Proposition 187 (1994) illustrated how quickly health care for immigrants can become a contentious public policy issue emerging from nativist sentiments. It heavily influenced the federal Personal Responsibility and Work Opportunity Reconciliation Act (PRWORA) of 1996, which to this day restricts even legal immigrants' access to medical and other social services. Although intended to be a broad and sweeping welfare reform, it contained such specific provisions to limit access to medical care to unauthorized migrants that it was initially conceptualized as *de facto* immigration policy (Fairchild 2004). The PRWORA and the Illegal Immigration Reform and Immigrant Responsibility Act, both passed in 1996, "created an environment in which immigrants are often ineligible, discouraged or frightened from obtaining public health insurance coverage and health care services" (Hagan et al. 2003: 459). Today, PRWORA legislation continues to deny social services to all legal immigrants in the U.S. for at least five years of residency, and unauthorized migrants are ineligible for any benefits at all (other than emergency Medicaid).

Policies requiring individuals to provide evidence of immigration status have immediate repercussions on access, based on research following such policy shifts in the U.S. For instance, Proposition 187 in California, which prevented undocumented immigrants from accessing publicly funded health care services, resulted in people delaying or discontinuing medical care altogether (Asch et al. 1998; Berk & Schur 2001). Similarly, after the passage of the Alabama Taxpayer and Citizen Protection Act, which required proof of citizenship, immigrants were less likely to utilize health care, even if they were exempt from the law's residency requirements. The passage of Arizona Senate Bill 1070 gave police the power to detain individuals who could not verify citizenship; as a result, individuals and families were less likely to seek out care, in addition to reporting increased anxiety about, and lack of trust in, law enforcement. This led many to severely restrict their mobility, which also impacted their overall health status. In Texas, immigrant health was affected by aggressive immigration enforcement linked to the passage of Senate Bill 4, which allows local law enforcement officers to investigate the legal status of those they detain.

In the U.S., health care remains conceptualized as a scarce and limited good, and there is no acknowledged "right" to health or medical treatment – even for many citizens, let alone migrant populations (Chavez 2003). Despite popular rhetoric, there is also little evidence that migrants are heavy users of public hospital systems in the U.S., where emergency rooms are easily overburdened as the only "safety valve" for uninsured persons. Although all indigent patients have access to emergency Medicaid services, which reimburse hospitals for emergency care of the poor regardless of legal status, unauthorized migrants' use is lower when compared to other residents (Berk et al. 2000). Beyond emergency services, the availability of care for migrants varies from state to state, where policies "oscillate between liberal generosity and stringent rationing depending on the political economic climate" (Horton 2004: 475). However, even though the U.S. possesses a fraction of the social welfare benefits provided in many other nations, the situation can on some levels ironically be assessed as better for unauthorized migrants. Because there are so many U.S. Americans and legal residents who are uninsured (or underinsured), the system has often been able to accommodate unauthorized migrants with less visibility. In fact, the functioning of the U.S. health care system is predicated on notions of categorization and exclusion, in striking contrast to the universal health care frameworks. As Hoffman notes,

> this contradictory and patchwork system of care – official policies of exclusion and cutbacks coupled with tolerance of provision at the local level – reflects the nation's inability to come to terms with the realities of immigration and the health needs of undocumented workers.
>
> *2006: 243*

Looking to other examples globally offers the opportunity to understand some other broad patterns. In social health insurance systems such as those found in the Netherlands, Belgium, and Germany, compensation for medical services is on a fee-for-service basis, which means that proof of insurance must be presented. By contrast, tax-based comprehensive systems, such as those found in Italy, Spain, or the United Kingdom, allow for more flexibility. Spain, in particular, has created a legal framework for ensuring coverage of irregular migrants, and in Italy, they are able to remain anonymous while accessing care in the regular medical system. These "humanitarian" models contrast sharply with other "utilitarian" approaches, where only emergency treatment is provided (Romero-Ortuño 2004). Notably, these systems came under strain with an influx in asylum seekers beginning in 2015 (often referred to as the "European refugee crisis"); without swift and clear resolution of their legal status, many of these access procedures for irregular migrants shifted as well.

However, even purportedly universal health care systems with coverage for all residents frequently exclude migrants, illustrating that lack of access is a direct effect of the state's efforts at illegalization and criminalization. For example, in Germany, a much stricter policy environment combined with the country's universal coverage makes uninsured immigrants highly conspicuous – because they lack required insurance documents – and thus targets of increased scrutiny (Castañeda 2008, 2009). Legal residency status (but not national belonging) is a precursor for participation. Germany's harsh policy environment toward unauthorized migrants is quite unique in Europe (Laubenthal 2008) and is a combination of laws restricting most legal immigration and a distinct approach toward migrants already living in the country. Despite some positive signs in recent years, unauthorized migrants are not afforded adequate access to health care (Castañeda 2011). Although technically they are entitled to emergency medical services based on provisions in the Asylum Seekers Benefits Act (§ 4 and 6), even these reduced services are often unavailable, since the Social Services Office that handles reimbursements is required by § 87.2 of the Foreigners Act to relay information to the authorities, which may lead to arrest and deportation. This requirement to report remains the central barrier to medical care and has been extensively criticized for impeding access for unauthorized persons; a recent United Nations (UN) review about the state of migrant health in Germany (UN Economic and Social Council 2018) suggested the country should follow the example of the United Kingdom and discontinue sharing of health data for immigration enforcement purposes. Despite the nation's commitment to universal health coverage, medical care for irregular migrants is typically relegated to NGOs, which, as in many other receiving countries, actively provide services to those populations neglected by the state (more on this below). At the same time, due to the influx in refugees in recent years, Germany streamlined its processes and introduced an electronic health card for those who have applied for asylum. Nonetheless, concern about overuse of services remains a major point in the public debate, and initial and intermediate-term access to healthcare remains limited and controversial.

Thus, one of the most notable patterns is the disconnect between the principles of purported universal health care systems and actual experiences of access on the ground. In some cases, coverage for non-citizens has been reduced or even eliminated, resulting in paradoxes between humanitarian universalism and nationalistic discourses based on ideas of deservingness. For example, Costa Rica has touted its reputation as a country having "health without wealth," with integrated public health and medical care delivery systems, low levels of health inequality, and guaranteed health care access to all residents regardless of citizenship status. However, economic instability and high unemployment rates led to a rearticulation of their health care model, reducing care for those who cannot pay (Goldade 2009). In France, principles of universalism are undermined both by national polices and by the interpretations and negotiations by frontline providers (Hoyez & Thomas 2016). While there exists a notion of "right to health," one study (Larchanché 2012) noted that doctors refused care to as many as 37% of unauthorized migrants who already held privileges to state medical aid – which, in practice, ensures that they don't have access to care. Thus, a general trend across several countries is that legal entitlement does not correspond with access to care (Woodward et al. 2014).

Finally, it is important to note that access policies can also vary within countries. For instance, some regions in Spain have defied a government law that prohibits free care to undocumented migrants (Thomas 2016); five of Spain's 17 autonomous regions, including Catalonia and Andalucía, agreed to continue to treat undocumented immigrants despite new laws excluding them. In San Francisco, unique strategies defied the otherwise decidedly hostile national context toward unauthorized immigrants in the American health care system. There, local government officials created a more inclusive environment by explicitly separating legal status from eligibility to receive local public services and benefits (Marrow 2012). In Switzerland, according to current interpretation of policy, undocumented persons have both the right and the obligation to obtain insurance as residents of the country (Jossen 2018). Yet policies vary from canton to canton, with a few, such as Vaud and Geneva, adopting more inclusive services for vulnerable populations, including undocumented migrants. Funding for these kinds of special programs often requires significant coordination between local administrations, NGOs, and service providers.

Beyond Policy: Other Barriers to Access

As discussed above, eligibility for health care coverage, especially access to state-run health services, is significantly determined by legal status, as migration and health care policies intersect at numerous junctures. Specific structural constraints resulting from social inequality, poverty, and violence lead to disparities in income, living and employment conditions, working alongside other gender, race, and ethnic hierarchies. Additional obstacles to accessing health care include linguistic barriers, external constraints like lack of transportation, and lack of familiarity with the health system (Castañeda et al. 2015; Quesada et al. 2011; Thomas 2016; Wickramage et al. 2018). These should not be viewed as discrete barriers but as "webs" that create more complex challenges than individual obstacles alone (Heyman et al. 2009).

Ambiguous and rapidly shifting policies means that it may be difficult for migrants to know what specific forms of health care they are entitled to (Poduval et al. 2015). For many, the constant pursuit of health care is time-consuming and very expensive. Financial restrictions may play a central role (Bilger et al. 2011). Communication barriers may further influence their willingness to access services; in the South African context, the multiplicity of languages has been cited as a major barrier, alongside discrimination by health care providers (Vearey et al. 2017). Other intangible factors (Heyman et al. 2009) include racism, stigmatizing discourses, and prejudices that shape ideas about what kind of care undocumented migrants deserve to receive (Vearey et al. 2017).

Requirements to disclose immigration status is a particularly noteworthy obstacle, which has been shown to decrease the use of health care services, as people fear potential consequences such as detention or deportation (Hacker et al. 2015). In some places in the U.S., local jurisdictions participate in federal enforcement programs such as 287(g) agreements and the Secure Communities program, which foster information sharing with U.S. Immigration and Customs Enforcement and the Federal Bureau of Investigation. As mentioned earlier, Germany has a law that requires relaying information to immigration authorities as part of the process for reimbursing services utilized by undocumented persons, which may lead to arrest and deportation. These kinds of arrangements heighten the fear factor when undocumented persons are seeking care.

Spillover Effects of Lack of Access

Policies restricting or mystifying access have broad spillover effects on families, communities, and the general population. Multiple studies have shown negative impacts on the willingness of lawfully present migrants and/or those with citizen children to access services; in other words, these policies produce a "chilling effect" on entire households (Sommers et al. 2012). For example, in the U.S., despite citizen children's eligibility for benefits such as Medicaid and State Children's Health Insurance Program (like Veronica's children in the introductory vignette to this chapter), studies show that those with undocumented parents access benefits at a lower rate (Hagan et al. 2003; Huang et al. 2006; Perreira et al. 2012). Fear of deportation and avoidance of institutions lead some mixed-status families to limit or delay services for children (Abrego & Menjívar 2011; Yoshikawa 2012), or withdraw from programs altogether (Hagan et al. 2003; Xu & Brabeck 2012). Some parents fear that enrolling children in programs will affect future chances at regularization, including family sponsorship or naturalization. The variability in the public charge assessment – in which applicants for permanent residency status must prove they will not be dependent on the government – has led some families to avoid obtaining services for their children (Mendoza 2009; Park 2011).

As a result, in the U.S., children in mixed-status families are more likely to lack health insurance and a usual source of care compared to those from non-immigrant households. Parental immigration status is associated with lower health care utilization in children, especially the legal status of the mother due to women's role as primary care provider. The potential for variable eligibility to occur among siblings is associated with lower access to care for all and ultimately reduced household resources (Hagan et al. 2003; Hudson 2009). Stratified access based on legal status may lead to preferential treatment of some children as well as resentments and hierarchal relations within the family (Menjívar & Abrego 2009), creating dilemmas for parents who may avoid services altogether to reduce favoritism (Perreira et al. 2012). The effects of "illegality" of some family members extend to the entire social unit, even for those who are lawfully present, with one *de facto* effect being that citizen children may lose their benefits because of a family's mixed status (Castañeda & Melo 2014).

This can be conceptualized as a form of "legal violence" (Abrego & Menjívar 2011), since laws that protect the rights of some simultaneously marginalize other groups, leaving them unprotected and ultimately more vulnerable. This legal violence is another result of "deservingness" assessments, that is, the ways in which some groups, but not others, are considered worthy of health-related attention, investment, and care. Exclusionary effects on entire families can be read as incidental and unintended consequences of policy or as a deliberate effect of state power. These avoidances of health care institutions illustrate how notions of "deservingness" have become internalized and have a chilling effect that extends to U.S. citizens, in what Laura Enriquez (2015) has called "multigenerational punishment." The consequences of disparate health care access on lifelong health outcomes are largely unknown, although the cumulative effects of social disadvantage are well established. As a result, "the costliest consequences of unauthorized status will emerge later in the life course, as current generations of unauthorized parents, children, and youth move into midlife and older age" (Suárez-Orozco et al. 2011: 457).

A lack of health care access also has spillover effects on entire communities and the general population. This is of course most prominent in the case of communicable disease, where monitoring and adequate access to care is fundamental to containing outbreaks (more on this in Chapter 6). However, a critical approach compels us to look beyond reductionist ideas of migrants as carriers of disease and instead consider holistic notions of community health and well-being, which includes prevention of chronic disease, safe neighborhoods, and food security. Lack of health care access combines with a pervasive fear of detention or deportation (to which we will turn in Chapter 9) to negatively affect the psychological, physical, and emotional health of communities.

Health Providers as Gatekeepers, Street-Level Bureaucrats

When it comes to policies regarding health care access for migrants, there is the possibility for a wide discrepancy between interpretations and reinterpretations at the local level. Often inconsistent rules must be decoded, and the discretionary practices of health care providers allow them to operate as "petty sovereigns" (Karlsen 2016), charged with discretionary powers by the state but entrenched in ethical and practical dilemmas as they attempt to translate policies into everyday service provision.

One of the major obstacles for migrants is bureaucratic disentitlement, with numerous studies highlighting how health care access – including emergency care – is threatened by administrative exclusion (Jossen 2018; Larchanché 2012; Fleischman et al. 2015). Bureaucratic disentitlement refers to the "insidious processes by which administrative agencies deprive individuals of their statutory entitlements and infringe on their rights" (Danz 2000: 1006; see also Joseph & Marrow 2017; López 2005; Marrow 2011, 2012). In everyday practice, this may present as withholding information or offering misinformation, isolating people so that they are unable to help one another navigate unfamiliar systems, and requiring extraordinary amounts of documentation for administrative procedures. In doing so, this prevents the transformation of statutory rights, such as the right to health services, into tangible benefits. Generally, this gatekeeping occurs through frontline staff in offices and clinics (some might refer to them as "street-level bureaucrats," Lipsky 1980), who have considerable discretion in the day-to-day implementation of policy and programs. They can make the process more easy or difficult for individuals navigating complex health and social service systems.

In addition, health care providers may play a positive or negative role as "petty sovereigns" or "street-level bureaucrats." A critical perspective compels us to account for power differentials in clinical settings (Biswas et al. 2011; Huschke 2014; Larchanché 2012; Poduval et al. 2015), as medical staff can facilitate or hinder access based on their discretionary actions and decisions. At the same time, lack of knowledge on behalf of health care professionals, who may be unaware of undocumented migrants' entitlement to care, factors into everyday service provision. For instance, in Spain, studies showed how health care professionals were left with unclear and inconsistent information about what kinds of care they could deliver to undocumented migrants following a change in the law (Jossen 2018).

Access via Charity Clinics, NGOs, and Nonprofits

There are many organized efforts to provide medical aid to unauthorized migrants who cannot access treatment through regular channels. NGOs, nonprofits, and charity clinics often emerge to fill gaps in health care, as patients are pushed into a parallel system because of exclusion from the mainstream. A frequent pattern across many countries is a discrepancy between the legal entitlement to health care services and the actual on-the-ground delivery of care to migrants through NGOs and charities (Altenburg 2012; Bilger et al. 2011; Weiss 2015).

Humanitarian-based alternatives, like free clinics, are an inevitable outcome of market-based health care policy and constructions of deservingness, as they seek to fill the voids left by the state's failure to provide adequate services to marginalized populations. However, rather than anchored in policy, these efforts offer only short-term, improvisational remedies, often under the guise of sympathy and/or generosity. These forms of medical humanitarianism help provide care to sick or injured persons whose capacity to access services is restricted (Minn 2010). Returning to the example of Germany, despite the nation's commitment to universal health coverage, medical care for unauthorized migrants is typically left in the hands of NGOs or charity clinics, which, as in many other nations, actively provide services to populations neglected by the state. Since there is virtually unrestricted access to office-based medicine in the country, emergency departments in Germany have typically played a rather minor role in providing care, and most unauthorized migrants visit nonprofit or charity clinics that offer limited services for free or on a sliding scale basis. These organizations are not sought out by the general public and exist exclusively for the purpose of providing medical aid to the uninsured/unauthorized. At the same time, the activities of these NGOs could technically be construed as illegal because they "assist" the continued unauthorized presence of undocumented persons (Castañeda 2012).

These efforts are generally spearheaded by citizens as gatekeepers, relying on community networks and social capital (Huschke 2014). One study with undocumented migrants in Denmark highlighted the important role of receiving aid from Danish citizens as a central strategy for migrants successfully accessing health care (Biswas et al. 2011). In many cases, this aid is an act of solidarity performed at the site, or field of contestation, of medical treatment. As such, it challenges norms about belonging and political community, contesting formal citizenship as a precondition for political voice. It may even disrupt the meaning of citizenship through acts of citizens on behalf of non-citizens (Castañeda 2013). In these acts, or protests, against the privileges of citizenship, medical aid becomes a powerful form of dissent.

Alternative Strategies for Treatment

In addition to seeking out parallel forms of care through charity clinics, migrants with limited access to care turn to alternative strategies, including visiting emergency rooms for non-urgent concerns and borrowing other peoples' medical cards (Roura et al. 2015). Other strategies include self-medication, often relying on "left-over," salvaged, and potentially ineffective medicines from others. Some migrants may rely on continued contact and advice from doctors in their home countries (Biswas et al. 2011).

Finally, as formal systems fail to meet the needs of a large segment of the population, alternative and informal channels of care proliferate, including illicit medications, unlicensed providers, and home treatments. This may include the utilization of local dispensaries that offer spiritual, healing, and religious services to immigrant communities, such as *botánicas* in the US (Viladrich 2018). Yet without adequate access to care, chronic illnesses become exacerbated, specialty treatment is out of reach, and they are unable to follow up on conditions requiring medical supervision.

Conclusion

This chapter has illustrated how host country policies impact access to health care for migrants, with a focus on undocumented or irregular migrants. How these individuals are included or excluded is indicative of a society's willingness to consider them as "deserving" of medical care and treatment. Even in purportedly universal health care systems, migrants are systematically excluded due to bureaucratic disentitlement and requirements to report their presence to the authorities. Overall, there is a vast disconnect between obligations under international rights conventions and how access to health care is translated in daily practice. This can have spillover effects on others around them, including family members and entire communities, whose well-being may be threatened by the combination of lack of health care access and pervasive fear of detention or deportation. While there are many organized efforts to provide medical aid to migrants who cannot access treatment through regular channels – charity clinics, NGOs, nonprofits – these efforts offer only short-term, improvisational solutions and can sometimes translate into absolving the state of its responsibilities.

Chapter 5 will examine interactions once access issues are (mostly) overcome: namely, the clinical encounters between migrants and health care providers. Using a critical framework, it emphasizes broader socioeconomic conditions and the influence of structural issues even at these microlevels, especially those related to legal status and the health care system such as cost, poor organization of services, language barriers, and social isolation. In doing so, it argues that these often have a greater impact on medical diagnosis and treatment than social or cultural differences, offering some insight into solutions, ranging from various forms of "competency" trainings and policies, increasing diversity in the clinical workforce, and building "migration aware" systems.

5

THE CLINICAL ENCOUNTER

Twenty-three-year-old Gheorghe, originally from Romania, arrived at a charity clinic in the German capital of Berlin with extreme pain in a lower left molar. He had taken over-the-counter pain medications for the past week with little relief and was also given antibiotics by a friend who recently had them prescribed for a respiratory infection. Examining the man's mouth, the physician said, "Nice to meet you. What are you doing here in Berlin?" Gheorghe explained in broken German that he is working in construction. He has been in Berlin for two years and resides with his cousin and three other Romanian men in a one-room apartment.

Following a brief exam, the physician gave him a slip of paper with a list of addresses of dentists who could help him. The first one was a mobile van that provides free, basic dental care to the homeless. He should not go there, she emphasized strongly, repeating this instruction twice to make sure he nodded to understand. "They won't take you because you are from Romania." Instead, she points to the list of private dentists further down the page, who have agreed to lower their rates for self-pay referrals from the nonprofit clinic.

Gheorghe immediately took the subway to the first address of a private dentist; however, the receptionist told him the office is too busy and cannot see him. He traveled to the next office, where he faced a locked door because it is closed on Fridays. Finally, the third office on the list agreed to see him and scheduled him for Monday (three days later), telling him to bring 100 Euros. They will extract the tooth, they tell him, since a root canal procedure is assumed to be too costly for Gheorghe.

In many countries, nonprofit charity clinics and NGOs have established referral networks or offer low-cost/free care for migrants with irregular legal status who lack health insurance. Gheorghe and those like him are in a liminal situation. Over the past decade, Germany has seen an influx of EU citizens from newer member states, including Romania. Although legally present, many are not enrolled in health

DOI: 10.4324/9781003307532-5

insurance coverage in their home countries and thus uninsured when they arrive in Germany. However, their unusual status often leaves clinic volunteers and the physicians and dentists in their network confused, since they may erroneously believe that, as EU citizens, they have access to insurance and the full range of health care services. They are frequently refused treatment for this reason. This is why the mobile dental van refused Gheorghe treatment; they prefer to use their limited resources to tend to (domestic) homeless persons, often turning away foreigners via their internal policy.

But there is another layer of exclusion here. As the receptionist who collects patient information at intake handed Gheorghe's chart to the doctor, she rolled her eyes. Later she told me that he is "another one of these Roma, pushy and demanding." This uniquely racialized minority continues to experience complex tensions present through its long history as Europe's eternal outsiders, including those who are EU citizens with legitimate freedom of movement between member states. While there are great disparities in available data, the size of Europe's Roma population is estimated between 12 and 15 million people. They face everyday forms of exclusion both in their home countries and when they migrate, including unequal relationships in the labor and housing markets and difficulties accessing medical care.

Ethnic discrimination is both interpersonal and institutional, ultimately based on ideas of how "deserving" a particular migrant is. Racialized hierarchies of inequality, poverty, and institutional constraints all contribute to poor health among migrants. Gauging the structural reasons behind people's displacement is the first consideration in understanding their lives; for Gheorghe, residential and occupational segregation of Roma in Romania led him to seek out work in another EU country. But the processes of institutional, economic, and political marginalization continue after they arrive; this includes where they fit into the spectrum of deservingness. Inequities in the well-being of migrants are heavily determined by factors such as discrimination, employment in dangerous jobs, inadequate housing, and poor access to transportation and other resources. All of these are evident in Gheorghe's case. Discrimination in the clinical setting can be both interpersonal (treatment by staff) and institutional (lack of dental care for migrants).

Finally, this case highlights that dental pain is a major concern among migrants but is often overlooked or discounted in seriousness. Migration status, social class, and poverty become literally marked on teeth as a visible sign of inequality and suffering. In many clinical and health research settings, dental issues – and their accompanying pain and social consequences such as disfigurement – are discounted as less serious. At the policy level, oral health is not accorded the same importance as is general health, although it is a much more sensitive measure of the overall strength of the health safety net (Horton & Barker 2010). The risks related to poor dental health are accumulated during the life course, and while highly preventable, untreated they can result in lasting physical, psychological, and developmental damage and lead to lost productivity, worsened job prospects, impaired nutrition, additional disease, and even death.

Gheorghe's molar was extracted three days later, the new gap in his smile joining those from other teeth that had been pulled over the course of his 23 years.

The previous chapter explored health care access for migrants; but what happens once they get past the door of the clinic? This chapter moves beyond questions of access to explore what happens in specific settings, ranging from public health departments, doctors' offices, specialty care, and the emergency room. It critically examines the clinical encounter between migrant patients and providers. A diversity of populations in clinical settings creates challenges, and health systems and providers must adapt to meet these needs to avoid adverse outcomes for patients as well as systemic inefficiencies. Social scientists have long been critical of employing simplistic notions of "culture" and ethnicity, which ignores broader socioeconomic conditions that influence health (Carpenter-Song et al. 2007; Hunt & De Voogd 2005; Kleinman & Benson 2006; Manderson & Allotey 2003; Taylor 2003).

Instead, the situation is exacerbated by barriers in the clinical environment, including prohibitive cost, poor and confusing organization of services, language barriers, and perceived low quality of care. While cultural and language barriers between patients and clinicians are likely to lead to poor health outcomes, factors such as design of the health care system and a lack of understanding of migrants' everyday lives also play important roles. A critical approach emphasizes the structural barriers to care and experiences of discrimination that often have a greater impact than social or cultural differences (Fleischman et al. 2015). A critical perspective is necessary to focus on the systemic barriers to care and devise appropriate solutions, ranging from improved policies, various forms of "competency" trainings, increasing diversity in the clinical workforce, and building "migration aware" health systems. The key questions that this chapter answers include the following: What characterizes migrants' clinical encounters? How do we move beyond simplistic notions of cultural competency? How can drawing on critical approaches to the clinical encounter improve the care received by im/migrant patients?

Critical Approaches to Understanding the Clinical Encounter

While there is a tendency in clinical medicine to approach disease as residing in individual bodies and the result of individual choices, the field of social medicine recognizes the importance of larger social context. Like other critical approaches, it understands diseases as strongly predicted by factors such as income, race, ethnicity, immigration status, and place of residence.

While training in medical schools incorporates an understanding of social factors, attention to these is often "trained away" during years of clinical exposure. Students in their first year of medical school learn to take a social history as part of the patient assessment process, where they must be attentive to all aspects that may assist in a diagnosis. "As they transform their eyes, ears, and hands into sensors for detecting hidden causes of disease, they also learn to ask probing questions to illuminate patients' social contexts" (Stonington et al. 2018: 1958). These social contexts might include, for instance, pathogenic exposure to violence during the process of migration, or exposure to pesticides in the fields. Understanding these circumstances can drastically alter the diagnosis and therapeutic plan. However, as they reach clinical years of medical training, students learn to collapse social history into shorthand biobehavioral risks, such as exposure to tobacco or alcohol. This is reinforced by what they read in medical journals, where there is an

> assumption that in clinical medicine, the biologic and behavioral world of a patient's body is more important than the social world outside it. This erasure flies in the face of increasing evidence documenting the role of social forces in determining health, disease, treatment, and recovery.
>
> *Stonington et al. 2018: 1958*

Critical approaches to medicine attend to the robust, patterned arrangements of social structure that produce and maintain health disparities, particularly inequalities emerging from institutions, the arrangement of health care systems, and the everyday effects of racism, gender bias, and neighborhood segregation.

Language and Communication Barriers

One major source of disparities within clinical settings, especially in contexts of "hyperdiversity," is language discordance between migrant patients and their providers. Mutual understanding between patient and clinician strongly impacts how medical conditions are negotiated. Effective communication is central to the process of understanding and diagnosing illness, as it is to understanding explanations for its origins and instructions regarding treatment and follow-up care.

Language barriers between patients and clinicians are an important determinant of overall poorer health outcomes (Meuter et al. 2015) and can augment the stress patients may feel, result in lower levels of treatment or medication adherence, and even lead to errors in clinical practice (Bowen 2001). On the other hand, positive health outcomes are associated with a shared language between physician and patient or other forms of highly effective communication during the encounter (Adams et al. 2015; Traylor et al. 2010). Professional language interpretation, in particular, can raise the quality of care. Systematic studies have shown that use of professional interpreters is associated with improved clinical care when contrasted with ad hoc interpreters such as family members or untrained clinical staff (Karliner et al. 2007). Interpreters, ideally, are not simply "neutral" translators of conversation but should be active participants in the encounter. Their effectiveness relies on the evaluation of medical relevance of patient contributions to the interaction; as a result, interpreters represent yet an additional institutional gatekeeper for immigrants.

However, in practice, professional interpreters are often routinely lacking due to resource (financial) constraints as well as poor organizational preparedness. Providers frequently rely on informal interpreters such as untrained clinic staff or the family members of the patient (including children). These can lead to technical, ethical, and practical issues, as ad hoc interpreters may add, substitute, or omit information. They may also volunteer supplementary information or seek to interpret the clinician's statements for the patient. The use of informal interpreters can impact patients' expression of emotional concerns, with fewer cues translated by them, according to a study of Turkish patients in the Netherlands (Schouten & Schinkel 2014). They may not be proficient enough in either or even both languages (and, in the case of children, may not have the correct anatomical vocabulary) to adequately convey important medical information. This may impair diagnosis and treatment, often with additional clinical consequences. One study on the use of informal interpreters among Serbo-Croat and Russian refugees and asylum seekers in Ireland indicated that it results in significant additional work for the clinician, who must negotiate between the benefits of having a friend or family member interpreter present and the professional responsibility of managing the language barrier (MacFarlane et al. 2009). Clinicians felt that the use of informal interpreters was inadequate and left them worried, frustrated, and with actual or feared experiences of error and misdiagnosis.

Depending on the particular national or local setting, there may be a patchwork of policies and resources designed to alleviate communication difficulties in clinical settings. There is currently no standardized curriculum or universally recognized certification for medical interpretation; however, some independent associations have published guidelines and codes of ethics, and in many places, certifications programs are available (though they may not be recognized elsewhere). The role of the medical interpreter remains unstandardized and often undefined but is undergoing a process of professionalization. In recent years, the use of dedicated interpretation telephone lines and videoconferencing technology have helped increase the skill level and availability of interpreters. However, these are lacking in other ways as they are impersonal and may create an even more alienating clinical encounter.

Patient-Centeredness, Diversity Sensitivity, and Cultural Competency

A great deal of attention has focused on ensuring clinical encounters are sensitive to the needs of patients of diverse backgrounds, including migrants from different cultures. Decades ago, medical anthropologists argued that differences in the *explanatory models of illness* (Kleinman 1980) between patients and physicians can lead to barriers during medical encounters and result in miscommunication and difficulties in diagnosis and appropriate care. This may ultimately lead to disparities in referral and treatment patterns. For example, researchers have long noted intense emotions such as fear, anger, or *susto* (fright) to be an explanatory model of type 2 diabetes in some Mexican immigrant and Mexican American communities (e.g., Poss & Jezeswki 2002). This suggests that other approaches may be needed alongside purely dietary interventions to address people's ideas about the origins of and appropriate treatment of diabetes. The explanatory model approach suggests providers ask a set of questions during an assessment to gain insight into what is most important for patients in terms of their health, illness, and appropriate care. These questions include, for example, What do you call your problem? What name do you give it? What do you think has caused it? What does your sickness do to your body? What kind of treatment do you think you should receive?

A move toward ensuring the *cultural competency* of clinicians sought to bridge these explanatory models and effectively translate between different forms of knowledge (e.g., biomedical vs. "traditional") regarding health and illness. By the 1990s, medical schools, nursing schools, and residency programs in places like the U.S., Western Europe, and Australia began to require training in cultural competency. However, length, content, and delivery approaches of trainings continue to vary widely, with Thomas (2016) reporting that across the European region they range from two-day to two-year long programs. Many of these programs are premised on the idea that increased exposure to, and knowledge about, cultural groups would help medical professionals offer higher quality care and this can, ultimately, lead to reduced health disparities (Brown & Closser 2016). However, the term itself has never been consistently defined, and over time, trainings extended the concept to refer to cultural awareness, cultural responsiveness, cultural safety, cultural sensitivity, cultural humility, and cultural capability, among other terms.

However, translating the concept of "culture" has turned out to be precisely the main challenge in these programs. Without critical reflection on this term, trainings risk reinforcing ideas that people from other cultures are exotic or inferior, ideas which often still have a strong hold in the field of medicine (Knipper 2013). While there is no question that people from different backgrounds have different ways of experiencing and understanding health, illness, and disease, cultural factors are not always the primary drivers. A consideration of social and structural conditions is also required and can help divert these problematic assumptions.

The primary critique of cultural competency approaches has been that they oversimplify patterns through an inexact use of the "culture" concept. In fact, culture is not fixed or static but "a dynamic, ongoing process and an emergent product of human interaction" (Carpenter-Song et al. 2007: 1363). A focus on "culture" often readily becomes synonymous with race or ethnicity – based on historically entrenched ideas of differences between groups – which leads to stereotyping patients and obfuscates their heterogeneity (Knipper 2013). Because many – especially early – programs of this type emphasized the importance of specific knowledge about a wide variety of groups, the result is often a list of discreet cultural traits or practices held by presumably static, circumscribed populations. This approach runs the risk of reinforcing stereotypes, "as if entire societies or ethnic groups could be described by these simple slogans" (Kleinman & Benson 2006: 1673). It presumes some easily delineated collection of cultural features, along with the belief that changes in these features are uniform across populations and requiring "several major leaps of faith" (Hunt and De Voogd 2005) to assume that health beliefs can be inferred simply by knowing national origin or ethnic affiliation. This can result in assumptions on the part of providers, which in turn may lead to different levels of information or different referral or treatment patterns (Thomas 2016). For instance, providers have been shown to embrace "culture" as a simplistic explanation for patterns of unresolved pain among Latino immigrant workers in the U.S. (Castillo 2018); as a result, they may treat them differently. A more effective approach emphasizes "dynamism and flexibility as key dimensions of culture" (Carpenter-Song et al. 2007: 1364).

Another major critique of such programs is that they fail to recognize biomedicine itself as a cultural system, thus downplaying important power dynamics within the clinical encounter. During the training and socialization of physicians, the biomedical perspective emerges as the primary frame of knowledge, while efforts at efficiency mean that patients' voices – and lay understandings of their medical concerns – may be left largely unheard (Good & Good 2003). This is the impetus for the emergence of *cultural humility*, which requires health care providers to recognize their own cultural practices and assumptions in addition to actively eliciting the perspectives of their patients. Nonetheless, cultural competency and cultural humility "capture only the fraction of the social determinants of health that stem from patients' mental constructs and the meanings they ascribe to things" (Stonington et al. 2018: 1959).

Thus, what often remains lacking is attention to structural factors such as working conditions, environmental exposures, access to health care, and affordability of medications. To return to the example of the explanatory model of type 2 diabetes in Mexican immigrant communities as linked to intense emotions such as fear, anger, or *susto* (fright), attention to the role of immigration enforcement might be an important factor. Raids, checkpoints, and other forms of intense surveillance toward racialized populations cause intense stress for many immigrant communities (undocumented or not), causing and reinforcing these intense emotions. By focusing on "culture," structural factors that impede access to care and adherence to treatment are also obscured. Health providers frequently fail to recognize the migrants' social context outside of the clinical space: their feelings of safety, working stressors, housing conditions, and food security. Social and economic features of the health care system, in addition to "subtle cultural factors" inherent to biomedicine, may prevent medical professionals from seeing and accounting for the social determinants of health of their migrant patients (Holmes 2012). Beyond oversimplifying their lives, an uncritical focus on cultural competency neglects structural factors that are more likely to result in health inequalities and patient outcomes (Carpenter-Song et al. 2007; Metzl & Hansen 2014).

Structural Competency in the Clinic

A call for "structural competency" (Metzl & Hansen 2014) has emerged as an alternative way of training clinicians to consider "the continuum of violence located in ethnic and citizenship hierarchies and international policies that place their patients in injurious conditions in the first place" (Holmes 2013: 153). As the authors of the *NEJM* social medicine series note,

> It may never be possible for physicians to become fully competent in as slippery a concept as "culture." But adding a basic competency in understanding how social forces affect our patients' health can help physicians to find more opportunities to intervene on their behalf.
>
> *Stonington et al. 2018: 1959*

Often, structural factors of poverty and powerlessness are the root causes of health in marginalized populations, including immigrants (Bourgois & Schonberg 2009; Farmer 2001; Kleinman & Benson 2006; Lock & Nguyen 2018). However, socialization practices in medical training, alongside economic pressures in health care systems, keep medical professionals from seeing the social factors that impact their migrant patients. "These barriers lead clinicians inadvertently to blame their patients – specifically their biology or behavior – for their suffering" (Holmes 2012: 879). Physicians may unintentionally perpetuate violence by ignoring socio-political and historical contexts. Without critical approaches included in their education, health providers will continue to use neoliberal understandings of health to reduce individuals to their biology, and this will influence their care and treatment (Premkumar et al. 2016). Thus, recent critical approaches in medical education have begun to emphasize the upstream fundamental causes of illness (Reich et al. 2016), and have sought to emphasize the influence of social, political, and economic factors on health outcomes (Neff et al. 2017).

Health "Literacy," Health Care Navigators, and Cultural Mediators

Even when language or cultural factors are not barriers (or can be readily overcome), migrant patients may still be unfamiliar with the health care system itself. The term "health literacy" is defined as an individual's capacity to access, interpret, and understand health information along with follow-up management of care (including medication use or referrals to specialists) to make informed decisions regarding their health (Nielsen-Bohlman et al. 2004).

However, this concept also places emphasis on the knowledge, skills, and behaviors of the individual patient, rather than on structural aspects of the encounter. Measures to assess such "literacy" have been predominantly developed with little but cosmetic input from patients themselves (Guzys et al. 2015). Nonetheless, there is value in helping migrant patients navigate complex health care processes in host countries; even people who have lived somewhere for a long time may benefit from guidance and support. Cultural mediation – a very wide-ranging and diverse field – can help in scenarios where patients are unfamiliar with the medical system or to facilitate interactions between patients and providers, going beyond the issue of language dissonance to address other kinds of miscommunication.

Community health workers (*promotoras*) represent one common form of mediator, strengthening communication between patients and providers and linking underserved populations, including migrants, to health resources (Logan 2022).

Community health workers are uniquely qualified as "connectors" because they generally come from the same communities in which they work, sharing a similar background and able to understand the social context of the people they serve. They can identify the health needs of immigrant populations and develop interventions based on those needs (Cupertino et al. 2013). However, the availability of these kinds of navigators is widely impacted by resource constraints and entrenched organizational practice, and there is little standardization across the profession.

Diversity in the Clinical Workforce

Encouraging diversity in the health care workforce – that is, ensuring that people of all races, ethnicities, sexual orientations, genders, religions, and class backgrounds are represented – is another remedy to better attend to migrants and other underserved populations in clinical settings.

Attempts to achieve, for example, "ethnic resemblance" between the provider and the migrant patient presumes that shared backgrounds will increase trust and mutual understanding. Indeed, some studies indicate that, when given a choice, patients in minority groups are more likely to select health professionals from a similar background as their own. They also report higher satisfaction with care in these cases (Mladovsky et al. 2012). On the other hand, some studies also show the opposite: that people *avoid* providers with similar background since they may have shared social ties in the same community. This may be seen as impacting the privacy of the patient or may heighten concerns around stigma and the emergence of rumors. One study in the U.S. found that Latinx patients were actually more likely to report "being treated with disrespect" in a racially concordant encounter with a health care provider than in a non-concordant one (Blanchard et al. 2007). And in a systematic review of 27 studies, only 9 demonstrated positive outcomes in race concordant relationships (Guzys et al. 2015).

Thus, the evidence is complicated, and further studies are necessary. While it is best not to assume that this is a solution in every situation, training and hiring a diverse workforce remains an important remedy.

"Migration Aware" Whole System Approaches

Scholars have also called for health systems, overall, to become "migration aware" (Wickramage et al. 2018) or "mobility competent," in the terms of the IOM. These more recent strategies to better serving migrant patients have focused on the concept of "whole organization approaches," such as those adopted in Europe to create migrant-friendly hospitals or in the European Health 2020 policy framework (Thomas 2016). These efforts conceptualize the provision of culturally competent health care as a task for organizations and systems, rather than focusing solely on individuals, and are more in alignment with a critical approach than is a focus on the behaviors and culture of individual patients.

Conclusion

While this chapter cannot cover all creative attempts to addressing diversity in clinical settings to improve encounters with migrant populations, it has pointed to several contemporary approaches and argued for the move away from individual-based understandings and toward a focus on structural factors that are more likely to result in health inequalities. While cultural and language barriers between patients and clinicians are likely to lead to poor health outcomes, other factors such as design of the health care system and a lack of understanding of migrants' everyday lives also play important roles. A critical perspective can point to potential solutions in changes to medical education, training to become more "structurally aware," and the development of migration-aware health care systems.

The next chapter, Chapter 6, examines the relationship between human mobility and communicable disease, a fraught topic that has received renewed attention in the wake of a recent pandemic. The linkage between migrants and infection is often exaggerated and has led to appalling consequences, yet it offers important theoretical and practical insights from a critical perspective, illustrating the persistence of colonial legacies, stigma for migrant communities, and xenophobic political responses related to border controls and limitations on movement.

6

COMMUNICABLE DISEASE

Amadou, a 31-year-old man from Senegal, dropped a few cubes of sugar into his tea, stirred, and lit a cigarette. He told me with wide earnest eyes, "There is no work now, because of the virus." He was happy to get out of the crowded apartment he shared with six other men in Casablanca, especially since the government curfews implemented due to COVID-19 meant he could not even leave the building after 9:00 p.m. Violating lockdown could result in up to three months' imprisonment and a fine of 300–1,300 Moroccan dirhams (about US$30–132). "Some Moroccans think *Sénégal* are more infected, you know. They pull up their masks when they pass me." He took a long drag on his cigarette and looked out into the bustling street, where people rushed to shop before curfew. "It's like with Ebola, they think we are bringing the disease." He was referring to the lasting stigma and impact of the Ebola crisis, when Morocco snubbed the rest of the continent by refusing to host the African Cup of Nations football tournament, citing the outbreak in three West African countries. For all the talk of "African brotherhood," Morocco, like its North African neighbors, has a complicated relationship with nations south of the Sahara.

While significant attention has focused on sub-Saharan Africans attempting to reach Europe, large populations unable or unwilling to return to their home countries are now settling in Morocco with irregular status. An estimated 700,000 sub-Saharan Africans resided in Morocco prior to the pandemic, primarily from West and Central Africa, especially Côte d'Ivoire, Senegal, Cameroon, Guinea, the Democratic Republic of Congo, and Mali (El Ghazouani 2019; Mourji et al. 2016). While the government has begun to address this new pattern of settlement – primarily in the form of nascent integration programs and the management of mobility across Moroccan territory – sub-Saharan Africans continue to live in precarious conditions around the country and face everyday racism, violent attacks, infringement of rights, dire poverty, and a systematic lack of adequate work opportunities. Most rely on the informal economy to make a living. Job market limitations force

DOI: 10.4324/9781003307532-6

them into construction, call centers, the service industry, or domestic labor; many face workplace exploitation and low monthly wages.

This precarity has been greatly exacerbated by the effects of the pandemic. Migrants like Amadou ended up deprived of work opportunities as well as access to aid, struggling to make ends meet under COVID-19 restrictions. Morocco imposed strict lockdown and confinement measures, which led to social tensions and stand-offs between young people and the police, particularly in Casablanca. While the government dispensed financial aid to informal sector workers who lost their jobs because of the crisis, no such steps were taken for migrants. Instead, they had to rely heavily on solidarity within their own compatriot communities as well as the charity sector (Mekouaz 2020). During the pandemic, some NGOs quickly adjusted their programs and resources to support migrants (Babahaji 2020). Amadou told me that, rather than sending money back to his family in Senegal as he normally would, he had even had to ask his sister in France to wire him money to survive, something which he felt great shame about. Meanwhile, he didn't know of anyone who had actually gotten COVID-19; neither he nor his roommates had been sick: "It's just a big lie by the governments of the world. They want to make control, you know."

In Morocco, the issue of immigration has had lower political salience compared to many other countries. As a result, policymakers have frequently been able to introduce progressive reforms extending – at least, in theory – provisions to migrants in health care, education, and labor sectors. For instance, since 2013, migrants in Morocco – regardless of their legal status – have been able to receive basic health care in public hospitals. This comes as the country recognizes its shift from being a transit country to a destination and builds on its "international image as a forward-thinking country on migration" (Knoll & Teevan 2020: 13). However, social services are already stretched very thin. The pandemic exacerbated many political and economic challenges in North African countries, including Morocco, as they continue to struggle with youth unemployment, deteriorating public services, and a host of governance challenges.

A public health emergency the magnitude of COVID-19 was new for the contemporary Moroccan state. From the beginning, it actively included migrants in its outbreak response, with the Ministry of Health's COVID-19 website dedicating a section specifically for refugees and migrants, including an explanation of symptoms, transmission, risks, and treatment (although only in French). Nonetheless, migrants have taken the brunt of the economic downturn and loss of work opportunities. As Amadou explained, "It was bad before coronavirus, and look at us now how bad it is."

One aspect of migrant health that has traditionally received a great deal of attention is communicable disease. Human mobility has been a critical factor intersecting with disease mobility and contributing to the spread of tuberculosis, human immunodeficiency virus (HIV), COVID-19, and Ebola, among others (Wickramage et al. 2018). Preparedness and response in times of health emergencies is reliant on accurate information about population movements for monitoring disease progression, predicting future outbreaks, and allocating public health resources. However, knowledge on actual disease rates among migrants is frequently hampered by lack of data; surveillance systems rarely capture or disaggregate information according to migrant status, and, as we have seen, definitions of migrants vary greatly, hindering the identification of patterns.

Communicable disease trends vary widely depending on the specific disease in question and are confounded by the heterogeneity of migrant populations (Williams et al. 2016). Nonetheless, as this chapter illustrates, associations between migrants and disease have resulted in stigma and discrimination, often built on legacies of colonialism. The key questions that this chapter answers include the following: Are migrants at higher risk of specific communicable diseases? How do legacies of colonialism play into communicable disease, including discourses of the diseased "other," stigma against certain populations, and the closure of borders to separate citizens from "foreigners?" What unique insights about migrant health can we gain by examining the trajectory of well-studied historical cases, such as tuberculosis or HIV? What was novel about the recent pandemic of COVID-19?

Critical Approaches to Understanding Communicable Disease

While migrants are generally healthy compared to native populations, as discussed in Chapter 2, the pathways through which they become at higher risk for communicable disease are complex and frequently linked to their socioeconomic position in host countries. It appears that some of the most consequential risks emerge after arrival, even if they come from countries with inadequate disease prevention and control practices, including suboptimal rates of vaccination for childhood diseases (Williams et al. 2016), or their risk is impacted by factors associated with the journey. In "host" countries, they often face living and working conditions that contribute to greater susceptibility. Many analyses have also failed to consider socioeconomic disadvantage and poor access to health care and prevention efforts on the acquisition or progression of communicable disease. And while it is a compelling topic, a myopic focus on communicable diseases in migrant populations runs the risk of overlooking their other important health concerns.

A critical approach to communicable disease is carefully attentive to the underlying structural causes of inequality. These may include working conditions, crowded housing, or poor access to food, all of which foster the conditions in which viruses or bacteria are easily spread. They may also include various kinds of bordering practices, which may lead people to take greater risks, or inadequate policy responses that marginalize non-citizens.

Legacies of Colonialism: The Diseased "Other," Border Controls, and Stigma

Colonial legacies have led to historical portrayals of migrants as diseased "others," who bring in dangerous pathogens and threaten the health of "native" populations.

This is evident in both the impulse to selectively close borders during outbreaks, as well as in the knee-jerk stigmatization of migrants and ethnically "other" populations as vectors of disease. These prevailing assumptions about migrants as introducing or spreading disease continue across the globe, resulting in the marginalization of "foreigners" as the politics of citizenship play out, blaming them for disease and denying them health resources (Amon & Todrys 2008; Grove & Zwi 2006; Harper & Raman 2008).

Even though international borders have closed in response to pandemics throughout history, the states of exception that accompany these closures also tend to precipitate new exercises of state power. In addition, these practices often divert resources away from critical public health interventions. Stemming disease was a major justification for border controls stretching at least as far back as the 14th century. During the Black Death, Italian city-states closed borders to contain the bubonic plague, issuing passes to travelers and imposing an isolation period of 40 days for incoming ships (bringing us the term "quarantine"). From this time forward, restrictions on travel and trade emerged as a primary policy tool against the spread of communicable disease. This was the case even when it was ineffective, such as during yellow fever outbreaks in the U.S. and France beginning in 1790s; these were mosquito-borne illnesses and thus not particularly responsive to border closures. In many places, the military was given authority over disease outbreaks, prioritizing border controls and quarantine throughout the 20th century and introducing securitization narratives to accompany them.

Simultaneously, increasingly strict immigration policies and practices in many countries, ranging from denial of access to invasive bodily inspections, have been rationalized as communicable disease prevention. Indeed, many of the current means of addressing outbreaks are inherited from the 19th century's preoccupation with border controls, which history tells us is a failed strategy (McCoy 2020). While restrictions on travel can stop outbreaks in the early stages of a pandemic, a focus on border control can also represent a diversion of investment in basic health infrastructure and preventive practices. History offers important lessons: border controls in response to crises tend to become permanent, with new infrastructures and regulations persisting well after their initial intended purpose (after all, the enforcement of the quarantine period in maritime practice persisted for centuries after the plague subsided).

The stigmatization of particular communities has historically been an element of discourse circulating about communicable disease, with immigrants often playing the role of scapegoat in the popular imagination, cementing wider cultural stereotypes. In this "politics of otherness," migrants are viewed as importers of disease and – along with other minority populations – a source of infection. Faced with the loss of control, particular ideas are often ascribed to groups regarding their increased susceptibility to communicable disease. As a result, "people faced with the threat of an illness … can deny their vulnerability by finding others to construct as its fitting targets" (Joffe & Haarhoff 2002: 968). Public reaction frequently leads to scapegoating and reinforcement of racism during outbreaks. U.S. reaction to Haitian immigrants during the first years of the acquired immunodeficiency syndrome (AIDS) epidemic – widely considered vectors of HIV during the 1980s – included measures such as deportation and incarceration (Farmer 2003), and the 2004 SARS epidemic was similarly linked to aberrant behaviors practiced by foreigners, particularly Chinese immigrants (Eichelberger 2007). Anti-immigrant rhetoric during the COVID-19 pandemic enabled public harassment and discrimination targeting certain groups, including, again, Chinese immigrant communities. These reactions are rooted in historical factors in a "complex web linking xenophobia and racism," along with a particular understanding of the "other" (Farmer 2003: 66).

Tuberculosis: "Penalty" for the Ruthless Exploitation of Labor

Tuberculosis is a particularly salient example that can underscore these practices of exclusion but also challenge popular understandings of the relationship between migration and communicable disease. It is estimated that one-third of the world's population is infected with the *Mycobacterium tuberculosis* bacillus (WHO 2021). Epidemiological gaps between high- and low-incidence countries are easily bridged when significant cohorts of migrants relocate, and it is among migrant populations that drug-resistant tuberculosis rates are the highest (WHO 2021). However, the proportion of foreign-born cases varies widely, with country of origin strongly impacting prevalence among migrants (Williams et al. 2016). While there have been declining trends in overall incidence in many countries, the proportion of cases in foreign-born populations has been increasing steadily in places like the U.S. and Western Europe (Gushulak & MacPherson 2000). At the same time, there does not appear to be increased risk for the general population, likely due to low levels of social mixing (e.g., cohabitation) with migrant groups.

A reemergent disease with a long history associated with poverty and deprivation, tuberculosis has been called "the first penalty that capitalistic society had to pay for the ruthless exploitation of labor" (Dubos & Dubos 1987: 207). The disease disproportionately affects the poor, racial minorities, and immigrant populations, and continues to be a concern because of high levels of human mobility and the emergence of drug-resistant strains. The dominant biomedical explanation, introduced in 1882 by Robert Koch, still fails to fully explain why only some infections progress into disease. Social scientists have sought to understand the extrabiological factors that contribute to the development of disease in some but inhibit expression in others based on cultural, environmental, and politicoeconomic factors (Ho 2003).

The association between migration and tuberculosis is not a direct one, but the key factor appears to be the relative deprivation of migrant populations in host societies and the resulting adverse effects on general health and well-being (Carballo & Nerukar 2001; Kistemann et al. 2002). Working and living conditions in the host country contribute to susceptibility, and limited access to medical care further exacerbates the situation (Carballo & Nerukar 2001). Even with initial screening for cases, many immigrants remain at higher risk for tuberculosis up to five years after entering the host country because of conditions of poverty and social inequality (Coker 2004; Jackson 2003). Multifactorial models are needed to better understand the complexities of the disease to deal with the "analytical challenge … to combine an understanding of the diversity of local contexts for disease transmission with a wider intellectual framework engaged with processes of global economic and political change" (Gandy & Zumla 2002: 392).

HIV/AIDS: From Stigma to Specific Vulnerabilities for Migrants

There is a complex and contested relationship between HIV and migration, with increasingly better insights today compared to the early days of the epidemic. HIV has long been considered a moral rather than biological disease of "the other," with immigrants heavily stigmatized in several settings. For example, in the U.S. in the 1980s, the early days of the disease, authoritative narratives often referred to it as the "4H disease," lumping together marginalized populations as particularly high risk: Haitians, homosexuals, heroin users, and hemophiliacs. This stigma toward Haitian migrants has been further upheld by imaginaries of them as harbingers of disease and disorder, so that "it is hard to overstate the extent to which Haitians as a collective have been blamed for bringing HIV to the United States" (McSwiggin 2017: 716), along with the resulting discrimination this community has faced.

While this stigma and discrimination against migrant populations with HIV persists to this day, there has been an increasing recognition of structural determinants and drivers of the disease since the 1980s, including social, political, and economic factors that affect prevention and access to treatment. Migration alone does not offer much explanation for HIV epidemiology, because associations at the individual level do not bear out at the population level. However, it does drive some aspects of the disease progression, such as treatment seeking and adherence.

Migration appears to increase vulnerability to the virus for both people who migrate and partners remaining behind (Anarfi et al. 2005; Banati 2007; Lurie 2006; Lurie et al. 2003). Migrants from regions with high HIV prevalence rates are disproportionally affected by the virus, when compared to native populations or other migrant groups (Williams et al. 2016). However, rather than simply being a migrant, various migratory processes are associated with specific vulnerabilities to HIV. These are sometimes contradictory; for example, common assumptions around risks introduced by the forced migration of refugees and asylum seekers have been challenged, with insufficient data to support claims that displacement increases incidence of disease or contributes to the spread of the virus (Spiegel 2004; Spiegel et al. 2007).

Southern Africa, in particular, is associated with a range of migration types, including temporary, circular internal migration between rural and urban areas, in addition to movements across international borders (Vearey 2011). In rural South Africa, migrants are almost twice as likely to acquire HIV when compared to non-migrants and controlling for other factors (Bärnighausen et al. 2007). However, the bidirectionality of infection is frequently overlooked, with studies showing those who stay behind – usually a female partner – also experiencing increased vulnerability to HIV because of the migration process (Lurie 2006; Lurie et al. 2003). These kinds of findings challenge dominant assumptions that HIV is primarily transmitted through male labor migration, where they are assumed to be exposed to the virus abroad (either internationally or in urban settings), with partners becoming infected after they return home.

Despite this complicated relationship, to continue with the well-studied example of South Africa, a range of inaccurate assumptions about the significance of migration endure. Although numbers of international migrants in South Africa are actually quite low, there persists a public perception that it is a much greater phenomenon than it is. As a result, there are many assumptions linking mobility with disease and the notion that migrants place heavy burdens on public health systems. International migrants are frequently represented as carriers of disease threatening the health of the host population, especially marked with the advent of HIV in the region (Amon & Todrys 2008; Grove & Zwi 2006; Harper & Raman 2008; Worth 2006). Furthermore, although public sector antiretroviral treatment (ART) is available free of charge in South Africa, discourse persists claiming that migrants are non-adherent to medication regimens, in addition to the notion that free treatment will result in additional "floods" of migrants seeking ART. As a result, in South Africa, increasingly xenophobic and even violent sentiments toward migrants have added to the problematic conflation of health and citizenship when it comes to HIV treatment (Vearey 2016).

HIV offers another illustrative example of the perils of focusing on individual choices rather than structural causes. As in other cases, infection frequently occurs in the host country, not the country of origin, and is often the result of circumstances that increase risk to specific disease, such as poor labor or housing conditions. Hardships related to migration status (e.g., lack of residence permit or economic resources) further affect the availability to health-protective resources. To illustrate this further, consider that sub-Saharan African migrants living in the EU remain one of the groups most affected by HIV. However, these rates are not only due to a high prevalence of the disease in their countries of origin but also due to infection after arrival in Europe. Studies in the United Kingdom, for example, note that at least 31% of sub-Saharan Africans living with HIV acquired it after arriving; a similar proportion (35%) is demonstrated for those living with HIV in France. Immigration-related hardships have been shown to increase HIV risks among this group (Desgrees-du-Lou et al. 2016). In addition to poor housing and economic conditions, migration creates occupational and social disruptions, including conjugal instability. These hardships may increase risky behaviors, including transactional sexual activity to cope with precarious legal status. Among migrant women, lacking a residence permit has been shown to increase casual and transactional partnerships (Desgrees-du-Lou et al. 2016). Women are especially vulnerable during periods without stable housing. As a result, structural barriers due to immigration policy are critical to understanding transmission and improving HIV prevention. Prevention strategies must recognize the role of gender and address migrant men and women differently, recognizing for instance that women lacking sufficient accommodations are more likely to engage in risky partnerships.

Most policy and programmatic responses to HIV still marginalize migration, even in cases where high levels of mobility are the norm (Vearey 2016). It is thus imperative to pay attention to the broader contextual factors affecting HIV management as they relate to mobility, such as treatment continuity and combination prevention approaches. Unfortunately, few countries have adequate systems in place to monitor HIV in immigrant populations, ensure that testing is easily accessed by migrants, or that testing is linked to appropriate treatment and care regardless of legal status. Migration should not be exceptionalized when it comes to HIV; otherwise, responses will fail to engage with the complexity and heterogeneity of populations and may instead seek to unfairly target them as "problematic" individuals (Vearey 2016). Responses must instead be "migration aware" and contain a whole-system approaches that normalize mobility.

COVID-19: Management of Human Mobility at the Global Scale

The COVID-19 pandemic fundamentally shifted the management of human mobility, and the immobility associated with it has been described as a "great disrupter" of migration worldwide (IOM 2022). COVID-19 has shown us the degree to which health across the world is interconnected, paradoxically at the same time as countries were preparing to implement the first-ever comprehensive agreement to improve cooperation on migration, the Global Compact for Safe, Orderly, and Regular Migration. As the pandemic unfolded, it laid bare just how existing social and economic conditions as well as political decision-making based on nationalist, xenophobic principles can produce unprecedented death and destruction.

Policy responses around the world included "stay-at-home" measures, school and workplace closures, restrictions on social gatherings, constraints to internal movement (e.g., via public transportation), and international travel control measures. The spatio-temporal propagation of the disease is highly related to mobility, with immobility through border closures, visa restrictions, quarantine, and social distancing the primary means for control. Immediate strategies against the virus involved a renewed emphasis on national borders, including the separation of residents from non-residents, in addition to increased policing and surveillance of already marginalized populations. COVID-19 abruptly halted the movement of people and goods via border shutdowns and travel restrictions implemented by hundreds of countries, some of which barred entry to anyone who is not a citizen or permanent resident, while others suspended the entry of people from certain regions of the world. One major result was the extended experience of immobility for many populations, as states of emergency declared in countries around the world forced people to face waiting and uncertainty. This extended beyond those typically conceptualized as "migrants" and included those who otherwise hold a privileged relationship to mobility, such as vacationers and business travelers.

While it may be true that diseases know no borders, "COVID-19 has once again shown that policy responses certainly do" (Ferhani & Rushton 2020: 458). During the pandemic, governments around the world implemented bordering practices that were in direct contravention to the WHO's strong preference for borders to remain open. The International Health Regulations (IHR) of 2005 were agreed upon by the member states of the WHO as a landmark form of global health governance – that is, by moving away from national self-protection and toward coordination to contain outbreaks – in the aftermath of SARS in 2003.

The IHR argued a clear preference for borders to remain open, weighing the overall goal of controlling cross-border spread of communicable disease with avoidance of "unnecessary interference" with international traffic and trade (WHO 2007). But the negotiations also outlined other specific reasons for maintaining borders as open as possible. First, evidence from other epidemics throughout history suggest that border controls are not an effective means of preventing communicable (and particularly respiratory) disease, buying at most a few days' extra time. Second, it is important to avoid non-reporting, as economically damaging trade and travel restrictions have incentivized governments to keep outbreaks secret in the past. This occurred in the case of South Africa, a country that immediately faced travel bans following its announcement about the discovery of the omicron variant of COVID-19 in 2021. Third, as the case of Ebola made clear, border closures can obstruct efforts at quick and effective response by hampering medical supplies and staff trying to enter the country. And finally, border closures were seen as having high potential for discriminatory practices and human rights abuses, including unjustifiable restrictions on nationals of certain countries, or according to, for example, ethnicity, religion, or sexuality (Ferhani & Rushton 2020).

So, what happened? Why were these recommendations largely ignored in the case of COVID-19? As critical border studies scholars have argued (Ferhani & Rushton 2020), the IHR recommendations were not "wrong" but rather inadequate to account for current global bordering processes, where a much broader understanding of "borders" is required. Much of the exclusionary bordering we find today takes place away from physical points of entry, and the IHR recommendations were heavily focused on these. For example, repatriation, evacuation, or "rescue" flights arranged by many countries to transport their citizens home very clearly produced exclusionary and discriminatory practices, but took place away from the physical border, enacted "not through policing of points of entry but through political decisions enacted via bureaucratic routines at 'virtual' national boundaries" (Ferhani & Rushton 2020: 475). These flights required coordination with other governments who had closed their air spaces and, while presented in humanitarian terms of "rescue," the stringent implementation of citizenship requirements revealed stratified preferences about who was worthy of protection, and who was not.

Thus, the widespread closure of borders and travel restrictions that were associated with COVID-19 were highly symbolic and have been called a "desperate expression of sovereignty" (Han 2020). Meanwhile, other bordering practices emerged, ranging beyond the country level and into communities and homes (Liu

& Bennett 2020), for example, through the introduction of mobile tracking technologies that enforce home quarantine, QR codes to track visits to locations, and vaccine passports. Nonetheless, discourse about the pandemic's role as a *security threat* to human health underscored border closures, travel bans, suspension of issuance of specific visa categories, and various forms of internal mobility controls including those that rely on tracking and surveillance technologies. As a result, it can be argued that the COVID-19 pandemic "ushered in alternative securitisation measures that would cause a shift in migration and security discourse from human-to-human aggression, notably terrorism, to the contagion of the pathogens like the coronavirus" (Byaruhanga 2020: 95).

And yet it is important to recognize that while borders closed during the pandemic, they did not fundamentally change. Rather, their violence has taken a toll on the same "disposable" bodies such as refugees, asylum seekers, and irregular migrants (Sterling-Folker et al. 2021). In both the external and internal bordering processes, economic, cultural, racial, and bodily differences continued to be negotiated, and "pandemic borders make existing mobility injustices more visible and deeper" (Sterling-Folker et al. 2021: 16).

As we have seen, migrant populations often face invisible struggles in the respective host countries in which they live. They frequently live in densely populated centers, where they have higher rates of susceptibility to diseases like COVID-19 due to crowded living conditions and exposure to mass transit systems. This may preclude physical distancing or make protective measures difficult. In many countries, immigrants make up outsize shares both of essential workers in the fight against the pandemic and those in the industries hardest hit by its economic impact. In the U.S. alone, six million immigrants work in frontline occupations, such as health care, food production, and transportation; another six million work in industries such as food service and domestic household services that have been economically devastated, making up 20% of the total workers in those industries (Chishti & Bolter 2020). They tend to earn less, lack health insurance, and be unable to take paid sick leave (or work from a home office), all of which negatively impact outcomes if they are infected. Furthermore, because of their legal status, they may be unwilling to engage with official testing sites or present to a hospital, even if their symptoms become severe.

In addition, many migrants, especially those who are undocumented or irregular, were excluded from government assistance programs that emerged in response to the pandemic, such as unemployment benefits or cash stimulus payments. Despite paying taxes for years in the U.S., for instance, many missed out on public assistance meant to help communities weather the pandemic. There were some exceptions that recognized the importance of aiding this population; for instance, the Irish government introduced a pandemic unemployment payment covering both regular and irregular migrant workers, and California allocated $75 million for Disaster Relief Fund for undocumented immigrants living in the state.

The constant surveillance and continued scrutiny of immigration status transforms public spaces into areas of risk of racial profiling and consequential deportation, decreasing the likelihood that undocumented immigrants will engage in a range of behaviors that typically keep them and their families healthy, such as walking their children to school, visiting outdoor parks, or obtaining essentials from the grocery store. At the same time, because of lockdowns, travel restrictions, and other social distancing measures, many of the most vulnerable immigrants were left feeling isolated from a social life that centered heavily on family and community gatherings.

Meanwhile, raids, detention, and deportations continued in many places during the worst days of the pandemic, despite the shutdown of other governmental activities. In addition to diverting resources away from tackling the pandemic, these actions promoted additional fear and discouraged immigrant populations from seeking out necessary medical evaluation or treatment. Following a highly criticized 2020 raid in Los Angeles, U.S. Immigration and Customs Enforcement (ICE) issued a statement promising that it would delay some – but not all – enforcement actions. Meanwhile, undocumented migrants staged hunger strikes in detention centers in New Jersey to draw attention to unsafe conditions and anxieties that COVID-19 would turn the facilities into death camps.

On a global scale, many migrants found themselves stuck in transit sites during the pandemic, caught between home and their purported destination when the virus erupted. Homeless and unfamiliar with the social and medical landscape, these groups were particularly vulnerable to the disease. Others live in crowded refugee camps where – as in detention facilities worldwide – efforts at "social distancing" are simply impossible. Finally, one of the lasting impacts of the pandemic will be that it may prompt new migration around the world, especially as people's livelihoods are affected and their communities flattened by the social, demographic, and economic impacts of the disease.

Despite travel bans and border closures, it has become evident in our world of massive cross-border movement that these are not particularly effective ways of containing communicable disease. While international travel restrictions were quickly enacted early in the pandemic – a time of extraordinary uncertainty as governments assessed the severity of the crisis – total border closures gradually eased over time (IOM 2022). Ultimately, prolonged border controls have proved to be an expression of national self-interest rather than an enduring policy solution. There is far more benefit to global cooperation than locking down borders.

At the same time, the COVID-19 pandemic prompted new calls for the regularization and inclusion of migrants. Resonating with protests against racial inequality and racism that gained momentum across the world in 2020, the important role played by migrants in critical economic sectors – agriculture, cleaning, delivery, or care work – has been magnified, and renewed calls for their inclusion emerged in many places. In France, for instance, hundreds of immigrants working on the coronavirus front line were provided with fast-track citizenship in recognition of their service.

Social exclusion and immigration-status precarity shapes the day-to-day experiences of migrants; the pandemic only further illuminated how legal status affects access to health resources and exacerbates pre-existing inequities. Their experiences have underscored existing insights on the production of social inequality while opening new ways of thinking about the interplay between migration and health.

Conclusion

This chapter has examined some of the key issues regarding migration and communicable disease through the lens of three specific cases: tuberculosis, HIV/AIDs, and COVID-19. In summary, migrants are often at higher risk of communicable diseases due to socioeconomic disadvantage, relative deprivation, and poor access to health care in the receiving countries. In addition, legacies of colonialism shape discourse about communicable disease and stigma against certain populations, particularly migrants. These public perceptions also underlie border closures and other attempts to separate citizens from outsiders using emergency measures that are often unfounded in public health science. This highlights the perils of focusing on individual behavioral choices rather than structural causes and systemic inequalities, and thus the importance of a critical perspective.

The next chapter moves to another topic: labor and occupational health. Many migrants end up employed in what have come to be known as "3-D jobs": dirty, demanding, and dangerous. This chapter uses a critical perspective to examine how these environments produce substandard conditions that endanger health and produce disproportionate rates of illness, injury, and disability, along with the lack of recourse for migrants built into legal systems around the globe.

7
LABOR AND OCCUPATIONAL HEALTH

These horses get treated better than we do.

These were the words of 30-year-old Javier, a groom I interviewed in one of the stables of a thoroughbred horse racetrack in Florida. Workers like Javier are part of an itinerant labor community following established paths of migration between tracks for the duration of the local season. Life and work on the "backstretch" – that is, the stable area behind the racetrack – is unique due to workers' shared mobility. In the U.S., the personnel required to care for horses is highly specialized by type of duty (exercise rider, groom, or hot walker), resulting in high levels of freelancing, in which individuals sell their labor to various employers without long-term contracts. Unlike other types of specialized labor, racetrack work does not carry high prestige, and these labor arrangements are often unregulated, dangerous, and characterized by informality, like many other forms of migrant labor.

Historically composed of members of the lower working class, since the 1970s this workforce has increasingly been made up of migrants from Latin America, primarily from Mexico and Guatemala. Many are unauthorized or semilegal, often having entered the U.S. without documents, violating the terms of their visas, or without proper work permits. Today, at tracks across the U.S., the language of the backstretch is Spanish, and small communities form around seasonal racing. At many of the larger tracks are temporary clinics, dormitories, churches, schools, and libraries set up to serve backstretch workers. However, at others, lower-status workers share small tack rooms in the horse stables as living quarters, and support is scarce. Everywhere, their pay is low, their jobs are dangerous, and few have access to adequate health care.

To learn more about health concerns behind the racetrack, my team and I administered surveys to those living and working on the backstretch. Predictably, the most cited concerns included injuries and pain resulting from working

DOI: 10.4324/9781003307532-7

directly with horses. This included musculoskeletal injuries, back pain, and overuse syndromes. However, safety regulations are widely ignored by employers, and injured workers are unlikely to pursue compensation they are entitled to because of their unauthorized status, language barriers, or lack of knowledge about health and legal services. Thoroughbred horse racing has changed little over the past century, which makes it unlike most other major sports, which have adopted safety practices and protective equipment.

Other health issues reflected the interplay between lifestyle and diet, such as high blood pressure, diabetes, and high cholesterol. The diets of the lowest-paid workers are often the result of financial constraints and the lack of facilities for food preparation and storage along the backstretch (no refrigerators or cooking because of fire risk) – opening a can of highly processed meals was often their only option. Dental problems represent one of the more profound unmet health care needs in this uninsured population. Finally, substance use – alcohol and other drugs – was common, which they attributed to their dangerous and high stress jobs, as well as boredom and isolation from family and the larger community.

All these health issues underscore the social and psychological impacts of inequality in the workplace and in everyday life, as well as significant barriers to treatment, including limited family involvement, isolation, low wages, and poor housing and work conditions. Despite their elevated risks, racetrack workers face numerous barriers accessing health care services, including language, location, transportation, and long wait times, and they often relied on already stressed segments of the health care system, such as emergency rooms. Most are paid below minimum wage and do not receive overtime payment as required by law. Living conditions are not always in keeping with guidelines for human occupation; living in tack rooms in the horse barns contributes to higher rates of illness because they lack electricity, running water, and cleanliness.

It is easy to believe backstretch workers when they say that "these horses get treated better than we do." The multitude of staff employed to ensure horses are healthy and comfortable is in sharp contrast to the dearth of resources for the well-being of the human workers. It is yet another case that highlights the health impacts of non-regulated, high-risk, and physically demanding jobs performed primarily by migrants (Castañeda et al. 2010).

The search for work remains a principal driver of international migration, amplified by global market pressures. This robust link between mobility and the search for work influences all aspects of life, including health, which makes a critical approach imperative. Most migrants end up laboring in what have come to be known as "3-D jobs": dirty, demanding, and dangerous. Race, ethnicity, nationality, gender, language, and legal status strongly determine the type of work they can access, and underlies the ways in which their vulnerability is heightened by exploitative labor arrangements. These environments produce substandard conditions that endanger health and increase risk for various forms of injury (Flynn et al. 2015; Holmes 2013; Schenker 2010). On a global scale, immigrants suffer from higher levels of occupational injury and fatalities compared with native-born workers in the same sectors. At the same time, they lack access to adequate legal, social, and health care services and face coercion, fear, isolation, and racism (Alexander & Fernandez 2014; Castillo 2018; Holmes 2007, 2013; Horton 2016; Kleinman & Benson 2006; Stuesse 2018).

This chapter examines the vulnerabilities associated with the work that migrants perform in host societies and the health hazards associated with them, as well as constraints to seeking recourse. It focuses on the risks and injustices associated with immigrant labor, as well as the barriers to seeking medical care and worker compensation. In contrast to focusing on individual choice and behavior, a critical perspective augments the scale of factors and employs the lenses of political economy and structural violence to understand how substandard conditions for injury and illness are produced (Benson 2008; Holmes 2013; Horton 2016). It also explores gendered labor patterns and the coercive conditions associated with trafficking and wage theft, to which immigrant populations are particularly vulnerable. As this chapter argues, the impact of workplace injuries and illnesses reaches beyond the individual to affect families and broader communities. The key questions that this chapter answers include the following: How do structural and systemic factors negatively impact the lives of im/migrant workers? What are the key theoretical frameworks researchers use to explore these issues? How does occupational injury foster negative synergy with medical care in terms of im/migrant workers seeking recourse? How does injury impact familial relationships and resources?

Critical Approaches to Understanding Labor and Occupational Health

The workplace represents a "convergence of the forces of the global macroeconomic structure and policy with the pursuit of survival and well-being for labor im/migrants, their families, and their communities" (Flynn 2018: 120). There are several international conventions in place for this population, in particular the International Convention on the Protection of the Rights of All Migrant Workers and Members of Their Families, a United Nations multilateral treaty from 2003. However, not all countries have ratified these conventions, and despite the commitment of those who have, enforcement is near impossible.

As a discipline, the field of occupational health developed out of a largely technical endeavor focused rather narrowly on the elimination of physical, biological, and chemical hazards in workplace environments. In doing so, until very recently it neglected the connection between illness and injury and their associated social phenomena such as class, race, and migration status. This was compounded by the bureaucratization of regulatory structures that systematically identify specific workplace hazards as well as the legal responsibility for mitigating injury and illness (Flynn 2018).

Structural approaches to occupational health can reveal how patterns of unequal health outcomes are the result of specific social arrangements (race, class, gender, immigration status) in interaction with particular job characteristics, such as low wages, non-standard work arrangements, lack of safety equipment, shift work, and outsourcing to subcontractors. Undocumented status is one major determinant of occupational safety and health (Flynn et al. 2015). In addition, type of work contract (permanent, temporary, none) plays a major role in determining health risks (Sousa et al. 2010). A recognition of the ways in which such social determinants impact occupational health is part of a larger trend toward understanding the central role of work in the overall well-being of individuals, families, neighborhoods, and populations. This more nuanced and holistic perspective breaks down traditional distinctions between work and non-work conditions, blurring artificial boundaries and countering reductionist approaches to better understand risks and develop more effective interventions (Flynn 2018; Peckham et al. 2017).

The concept of *structural vulnerability* examines workers' location in a hierarchical social order of disadvantaged persons and how this produces and exacerbates illness. As in prior chapters, this critical framing represents a necessary corrective to approaches that focus on individual behaviors or workplace equipment issues as the primary sites of intervention. In the case of immigrant workers, structural vulnerabilities include

> relationships between the intensification and consolidation of capitalist production and related management and state labor, criminal, and im/migrant surveillance systems, shifting political definitions and enforcements of deportability, and heightened risks and rates of injury, illness, and death amongst affected and afflicted workers all over the world.
>
> *Saxton & Stuesse 2018: 70*

The worker's body thus becomes a site for the expression of the disjuncture between welfarist and neoliberal rationalities, the target of a mundane disciplinary gaze that protects the employer's interest in functional bodies (MacEachen 2000).

Accurate assessments of occupational injury or illness (and deaths) are already hampered by inconsistent and often underfunded surveillance systems and reporting mechanisms. This is compounded when a person has migrant status, since these systems may be even less accessible to them or because they may be employed in irregular conditions without formal contracts. Additionally, they may not be fully informed about their rights, or may avoid reporting incidents due to stigma or out of fear of losing their jobs. Finally, occupational illness and injury compounds in the bodies of immigrant workers over the life course, often exacerbating or leading to synergistic interactions with other illnesses (Horton 2016).

Negative tropes about migrants further legitimatize and rationalize patterns of exploitation (Benson 2008). Often, migrants internalize narratives about their low worth – a form of symbolic violence – and this impacts their willingness to risk their safety, report injury, or seek out health care (Quesada et al. 2011). The concept of "faciality" can account for "how social power overlaps with perception to legitimize patterns of social subordination, economic exploitation, and spatial segregation" (Benson 2008: 589). Risk factors in the social and working environment, as well as access to rights such as paid sick leave, are closely linked with migrants' position in the social structure, especially for certain nationalities (Agudelo-Suárez et al. 2009). Ethnicity and indigeneity further stratify and increase structural vulnerability (Holmes 2011, 2013). For example, one study found that indigenous Triqui migrants from Oaxaca, Mexico were perceived by employers to be "too short" for picking apples and thus hired instead for picking berries. This stereotype was adopted by the workers themselves, who claimed that "Oaxacans like to work bent over," naturalizing their own ability to do backbreaking work that other migrant populations prefer not to do. Thus, "(a)ttention to what is hidden in U.S. agriculture reveals the segregation of labouring bodies by perceived ethnicity and legality into a hierarchy that, in turn, produces correlated suffering" (Holmes 2007: 61). These inequalities, in turn, "are effectively naturalized through the symbolic violence enacted by discrepant hiddenness of bodies, perceived bodily differences, ethnic concepts of pride, and imputed humanity based on body position" (Holmes 2007: 61).

Gender remains one of the fundamental social relations impacting immigration patterns, especially when it comes to labor. Undocumented and displaced women are more likely to work in informal economies such as health care, domestic work (including child care and cleaning), street vending, and the garment industry (Hondagneu-Sotelo 2001, 2003). Women in "pink collar" jobs have slightly more opportunity for upward mobility but still face various structural issues at home and the workplace. A study with Sri Lankan woman after they have returned home from working abroad as maids indicated that they suffered a variety of patterned abuses, including physical, financial, verbal, and emotional (Wickramage et al. 2018).

For those im/migrants who are undocumented, the *condition of illegality* itself is an axis of social stratification that works to produce pathogenic conditions (Cartwright 2011). For undocumented persons, legal status, country of origin, race, ethnicity, class, and gender combine to render their labor flexible and cheap (Cartwright 2011; Holmes 2013; Smith-Nonini 2011). The convergence of undocumented status, employment patterns, and exclusion through policy (e.g., workers compensation laws) produces an extreme vulnerability that can be characterized as a form of *legal violence* (Stuesse 2018). Their daily lives may be full of uncertainty and insecurity, especially as people remain vulnerable to the effects of deportability through immigration enforcement. All these factors produce a labor force that is easily viewed as "discardable," "disposable," or even as a form of "renewable energy" (Chavez 1992; Stuesse 2016; Smith-Nonini 2011). Migrants often report that they are unable to object to poor conditions, as they feel that they are forced to endure any kind of situation because of their legal status (Agudelo-Suárez et al. 2009).

Even with "legal" or authorized labor migration, abuse may occur throughout the recruitment process and in the workplace. For example, the kafala system (نظام الكفالة) oversees and manages migrant laborers working in the construction and domestic sectors in Kuwait, Lebanon, Qatar, Oman, Saudi Arabia, and the United Arab Emirates. This system of sponsorship ties migrant workers' visas to their employers, which can easily fuel exploitation and abuse. Employers have authority to grant permission for the worker to enter the country, transfer employment, or depart. In addition, a number of wage theft patterns have been found to relate to this system (Wickramage et al. 2018).

Occupational injury and injustices often act in synergy to worsen the effects of chronic disease, disability, environmental exposures, substance use, poor living conditions, and social isolation for immigrants. Already discussed in prior chapters, the concept of *syndemic* (synergistic epidemic) is a particularly useful lens with which to examine linkages between different health problems that interact with one another to create an excess burden of disease (Singer & Claire 2003). Another approach that recognizes how health outcomes are embedded in social lives is the *life course* perspective. Focusing on four main tenets – environment/place, timeline, timing, and equity – this approach illuminates how social exclusion structures one's time in asset-building or disadvantaged contexts, thus contributing to inequities in health outcomes across the life course and even over generations (Gee et al. 2012). In terms of illness, the concept of *chronicities* (Manderson & Smith-Morris 2010) breaks down artificial boundaries between acute and chronic conditions. In addition to urging us to not consider diseases in isolation, this approach points to how treatment is structured through political boundary work, which frequently isolates work-related complaints to a realm of their own with particular treatment protocols.

Occupational Hazards

In April 2013, a garment factory in Rana Plaza located in the Dhaka District of Bangladesh collapsed, killing at least 1,134 people, and injuring another 2,500. The deadliest garment factory disaster in history, the eight-story building collapsed because of structural failure. This incident brought to light the extremely hazardous working conditions in low-wage employment sectors around the world. Similarly exploitative conditions have been made public by production line workers at Foxconn in Shenzhen, China. These predominantly migrant workers are systematically excluded from public housing and forced to live in expensive, densely packed neighborhoods surrounding the factory. These cases exposed the broader public, if one for a few moments, to the unsafe and exploitative work conditions that many migrants face.

The risks of injury that workers encounter are highly predictable (Quandt et al. 2006). In many agricultural fields in which immigrant labor predominates, for instance, tasks are frequently structured through repetitive motion or continued use. Fortunately, this also means that effective opportunities for intervention exist, since changes can be made to prioritize the health of the worker over the efficiency of the task. This might include personal protective equipment to prevent exposure to dangerous chemicals, ergonomic improvements to workstations, and peer education programs (Arcury et al. 2012, 2013; Grzywacz et al. 2010; Marín et al. 2009; Monaghan 2011).

At the same time, however, workers – especially those in subcontracted or day labor positions – may lack training or experience with the tasks they are expected to carry out. This may be compounded by substandard or a lack of equipment altogether, or other pressures that lead employers to bypass safety precautions (Walter et al. 2002). A study of occupational injury among non-agricultural, urban immigrant Latino workers showed that relatively few received job safety training (often offered only in English), despite legal requirements to deliver information about workplace hazards (Pransky et al. 2002).

In many, if not most, informal labor sectors, such as agriculture and domestic work, migrant workers face highly unregulated conditions and may be unaware of their legal rights, if these even exist. In some nations, this is compounded by underdeveloped legal systems, corruption, bans on trade unions, as well as general fear of authorities, making legal recourse uncommon. Nonetheless, worker-driven efforts in a number of settings have been successful in negotiating better work conditions, filing complaints with government offices, and educating about labor rights.

Labor Abuses: Trafficking and Wage Theft

Immigrant populations are particularly vulnerable to coercive conditions associated with labor trafficking and wage theft, defined as the denial of legally owed wages and benefits. This can take the form of underpayment or outright non-payment for work completed but may also present as refusal to pay the minimum wage, denial of overtime or breaks, or various forms of job misclassification that result in an individual not receiving agreed-on or statutory compensation. Wage theft can be an indicator of more severe abuses like labor trafficking, which includes the use of force, coercion, or fraud. Most abusive labor practices, however, "fail to meet this high and explicit threshold [of trafficking] or attract law enforcement concern, which often tends to prioritize sex trafficking" (Galemba 2021: 94).

Critical approaches explore

> how individual legal remedies or criminal justice responses can risk obscuring the ways that wage theft is embedded along a continuum of legal and illegal exploitative labor practices that are normalized and maintained by the broader degradation of work and the criminalization of immigration.
>
> *Galemba 2021: 91*

Immigrants are especially vulnerable to wage theft – particularly if they work as day laborers in informal settings – because their marginal sociostructural position and often uncertain legal status lead to insecure work environments that predispose them to workplace injury, harassment by both employers and police, and other forms of discrimination. Increasingly, research has focused on how workers contest their victimization and locate options to recover unpaid wages (Galemba 2021).

Worker Injury and Injustices

Workers' compensation systems began in 19th century Europe during industrialization. Germany was the first to introduce a legal doctrine for employer liability, followed by several other nations. Contemporary worker compensation systems are often based on employer contributions to an insurance program (e.g., Western and Central Europe, the U.S.), while others are financed through taxes (e.g., United Kingdom, southern Europe, Scandinavia). In addition, a variety of mutual aid societies (or "friendly societies") exist around the world – some of them historically founded by migrant populations, such as the Martí-Maceo Society of Florida, started by Afro-Cuban immigrants – in which workers support one another collectively, protecting members from debts incurred through illness, injury, death, or old age, and providing aid to workers' widow(er)s and orphans.

Migrant workers have historically been marginalized by formal systems of aid. The concept of *workers' decompensation* can be used to describe the "multilayered impacts that federal and state austerity measures, workplace hazards, and anti-immigrant policies are having on the health and welfare of im/migrant workers" (Saxton & Stuesse 2018: 66). Different safety net systems and policies intersect and often contradict or counteract one another. While workers' compensation systems emerged following industrialism, when workplace injuries in manufacturing were frequent, over time regulatory rollbacks gutted the system. As a result, workers' bodies across the globe are now in chronic states of "decomposition." In medical terms, this refers to the loss of the ability to cope with excess burdens or stress, as is the case in organ failure or for chronic conditions like diabetes. Following a debilitating work injury, people often rely on other parts of their body to support them (shifting to use the other side, for instance). But they may also rely more on their family and personal networks for daily tasks or to generate income; these added roles can, in turn, result in stress to those around them, creating a vicious cycle of instability. Thus, social systems also suffer irreparable harm through the erosions of effective health and occupational safety systems. The concept of decompensation allows us to "visualize and analyze the multilayered effects of cut and rolled-back support systems, as well as the embodied consequences for immigrant workers, their families, and communities" (Saxton & Stuesse 2018: 66).

Three issues increase the likelihood of becoming injured: workplace conditions, employer insensitivity, and employees' lack of knowledge (Beardwood et al. 2005). Where rights and benefits are available to immigrant workers who become injured, there is frequently a lack of knowledge about these rights. They are less likely to file claims, which may be due to unfamiliarity with the process, fear of retaliation by their employer, or language and cultural barriers. Most severe work injury cases do not result in a worker's compensation claim, in part because of employer actions such as discouraging or threating workers if they file a claim (or simply not informing them about this coverage). On other cases, workers may not understand information due to language barriers or be reluctant because they believe filing may lead to job loss or deportation (Pransky et al. 2002).

Work-related injuries in many host countries are governed by a complex array of laws, insurance companies, approved health care providers, metrics of evaluation, treatment protocols, and compensation schedules. These may vary by jurisdiction, type of employment sector, and even by type of injury. As a result, workers' compensation systems are frequently "cumbersome, frustrating, and demeaning," adding to workers' already stressful experiences of illness or injury (Strunin & Boden 2004: 338). In many places, these systems have been made increasingly difficult for injured workers to access, effectively shifting the burdens from employers to workers and their families, non-profit organizations (including mutual aid societies), and taxpayers. Workers who do not follow predictable patterns of returning to work are often blamed for their own lengthy recovery, and any efforts to negotiate or have control over their case may be perceived as resistance (Beardwood et al. 2005). Challenges for compensation systems thus include "medico-legal issues, the potential perversion of science and medicine, and the danger of stigmatization of claimants" (Lippel 2012: 13).

Thus, migrant workers face multiple systemic barriers in accessing compensation systems, and while some of these are due to a lack of knowledge or inaccessible processes, employers may also have an interest in blocking claims. Migrant workers are more likely to face contestation of their claims than non-migrants. For example, a study of occupational injury and health care seeking experiences of migrant poultry workers in the southern U.S. documented the lengths to which employers go to avoid reporting and treating instances of workplace injury, ranging from obstructionist doctors and nurses in company settings, to retaliation and firing of injured undocumented workers (Stuesse 2018). Indeed, the workers compensation system has many failings as a medio-legal project that reproduces docile workers as an exploitable labor force. The concept of "temporality" refers to the "spontaneous and arbitrary imposition of strategies by employers as a response to situations in which workers attempt to bargain to ameliorate exploitation in the workplace or in response to workplace injuries" (Yea 2017: 179). Immigration enforcement policies and practices further produce anxieties in communities and can work to undermine efforts to promote worker health (Gleeson 2012). Migrant workers, particularly those who lack formal legal status, may not believe that they have a right to a safe workplace, even if those rights are formally extended to them.

The impact of workplace injuries and illnesses reaches beyond the individual to also affect their families and communities. Especially when they are unable to access support or compensation, their families may take up additional responsibilities to assist with recovery (Boden et al. 2001; Dembe 2001). Since work is often an important source of identity, an injured worker may struggle to adjust to the loss of their perceived place in the world (Saunders & Nedelec 2014; Stone 2003), an issue that is often highly gendered, especially if the male or female in the household is expected to be the "breadwinner." When work is a central part of their sense of self, immigrants may experience a significant disorientation and discomfort that can affect overall health. Those who cannot return to work can become caught in a vicious cycle, with financial difficulties compounded by family and marital stress, diminished self-worth, depression, anger, and substance abuse. In addition to further impeding their return to work, these issues can become more incapacitating than the initial injury or illness itself.

Demonstrating Deservingness and Legitimacy in the Medical Encounter

One of the primary obstacles to successfully being awarded compensation is that the process requires petitioners to demonstrate that their claims are legitimate and deserving, both of which can be problematic for migrant workers. The workers' compensation system inherently positions the claimant – the worker – as suspect, requiring them to prove their case. This is yet another arena where migrants, particularly those without legal status, face suspicion and stigma.

As part of the assessment of health-related deservingness, they may be forced to make various "legitimation maneuvers" (Quesada et al. 2011). Injured migrant workers must convince doctors, employers, insurance providers, and lawyers that they are "legitimate sufferers" (Jaye & Fitzgerald 2012). What is allowed to "count" as a work-related illness is often prescribed by reductionist biomedical metrics and culturally shaped ideas utilized by insurance companies and health care providers. Often, it must first be determined if there is a pre-existing condition underlying the illness or injury that can be partially blamed, thus allowing the claim to be dismissed. Furthermore, for certain occupational illnesses, there is often an unclear causal link. Horton (2016) demonstrates this in the case of heat stress and heat stroke among migrant farmworkers; the connections between the conditions of labor and the worker's ill body can be easily denied or rendered uncertain. As a result, it becomes easier for employers, insurance companies, health care professionals, and policymakers to place the origin and burden of recovery directly on injured workers (Grabell & Berkes 2015; Leigh & Robbins 2004).

Migrant workers frequently face barriers during clinical encounters when dealing with occupational injuries or illness. When physicians are positioned as gatekeepers to the worker's compensation system, it erodes the trust necessary in a patient-physician relationship (Castillo 2018). In an "ordinary" clinical encounter, a physician evaluates the patients' history, examines the sites of symptoms, and orders laboratory or imaging evidence to ultimately decide on a treatment plan; however, in the medico-legal framework of workers' compensation, this clinical interaction also serves the purpose of legitimizing the worker's claim to injury (Castillo 2018). The biomedical evidence and the physician's assessment thus supplants the patient's treatment needs as well as their own testimony, which is viewed as suspect. Injured workers, thus, are not trusted as it is assumed they have something to "gain" from filing a claim; an "objective" evaluation of the body through the physician's medical gaze is preferred as it allows for the social context to be rendered irrelevant until the legal system deems it necessary (Holmes 2013). By contrast, allowing patients' subjective experiences to speak would allow claimants' histories highlighting their structural vulnerability to be considered as part of legal proceedings (Saxton & Stuesse 2018; Stuesse 2018).

Assessment of pain by medical professionals has been found to be influenced by the national, ethnic, or racial origin of patients (Ernst 2000; Castillo 2018). Prejudice and bias easily emerge, and the medical literature is full of historical characterizations of migrant workers as somatizers or hypochondriacs, noting "migrants' uncontrolled, hysterical, and dramatic expressions of pain or discomfort" in several contexts (Castañeda 2012: 832). In Germany, for example, Turkish and Italian guestworkers' expressions of pain were described as "Mediterranean Syndrome" or even "mama mia syndrome," characterized by a lower pain tolerance than that of Europeans (Castañeda 2012; Ernst 2000). Physicians' perceptions of purported cultural factors also explain disparities in pain management for Latinos in the U.S. today; there are commonly held stereotypes about these patients' pain tolerance. As a result, they are more likely to be under suspicion for malingering or somatization. In fact, "The constant in these observations is not a specific immigrant group or host country, but instead immigrants' pain being perceived differently regardless of the cultural context" (Castillo 2018: 100). The ubiquity of this idea is a pattern across different health systems and national settings and highlights common responses to migrant patients. Language barriers between physician and patient can, of course, further exacerbate these issues.

Finally, while some workers recover and return to work, others remain with lifelong disabilities. Further legitimation issues may persist in cases where someone does not match a clear "template of recovery" (Beardwood et al. 2005: 31). For many migrant workers, light duty, reduced hours, and physical therapy regimens are simply not possible due to the nature of their employment; neither is taking time off in the hope of recovery and eventual return. This frequently has a major impact on participants' perception of themselves as hardworking, motivated people, which is made more difficult when employers or coworkers label them as liars, malingerers, or lazy (Jaye & Fitzgerald 2010).

> A striking and repeated area of concern expressed by injured workers was the lack of respect that they faced in the absence of any wrongdoing. Many felt compelled to provide evidence of their commitment and motivation to work to counteract the negative assumptions and stereotypes that they faced.
>
> *Beardwood et al. 2005: 40*

In the meantime, they may face social stigma and exacerbation of health conditions, in addition to threats to their identity and ability to fulfill prescribed social roles. As a result of occupational injury, some eventually return to their home country as disabled bodies, with disability and care essentially outsourced to their families and to lower-income nations more generally.

Conclusion

This chapter has examined the occupational health hazards migrants face, especially increased risk of injury and death, because of their marginalization and vulnerability to exploitative labor conditions. A critical perspective can help illuminate how substandard conditions for injury and illness are produced by structural factors. Migrants also subsequently face systemic barriers in seeking medical care and justice via workers' compensation systems. Employers may discourage or threaten those who file claims, and work-related injuries are often extraordinarily difficult to navigate. A primary obstacle is requirements to demonstrate that an injury claim is legitimate, and migrants must convince doctors, employers, insurance providers, and lawyers that they are legitimate sufferers. Immigration enforcement policies and practices can further undermine efforts to promote worker health. As this chapter has argued, the impact of workplace injuries and illnesses reaches beyond the individual to affect families and broader communities.

The next chapter moves to a discussion of gender and sexuality to amplify how these issues play into the study of migrant health. It explores how population policies are inscribed on the bodies of migrant women, with stratified reproduction highlighting notions of citizenship and belonging in various host nations. Gender is a fundamental social category shaping immigration patterns, producing major shifts in family structures, intimate relationships, and social roles. Sexuality is another landscape in which people contest and renegotiate the meanings behind citizenship and belonging, as the next chapter elaborates.

8

GENDER, SEXUALITY, AND MIGRANT HEALTH

Sarah arrived in Berlin from Ghana with next to nothing – just "two pair of trousers" – because she was not planning on staying. She had come with a group of women to explore possibilities for work. After three months, when her tourist visa expired, she became "illegal." At a party hosted by friends, she met Joaquim, a man from Mozambique who had lived in Germany more than 20 years. After a few months of dating, she discovered she was pregnant – something she hadn't planned. "Of course not," she told me,

> This is not the right time, when you're in Europe, all alone with no papers! In Africa I have my family, a lot of family who can help out. Before the baby comes, and afterwards, there are always people to take care of you.

A friend recommended that Sarah go to the Center for Family Planning, a non-profit organization that provides prenatal care for undocumented women in Berlin for a nominal fee. From there, she was referred to the Migrant Clinic (a pseudonym), which arranged blood tests and a low-cost delivery spot at a local Catholic hospital. In both places, she felt comfortable with the doctors. "I told my family that I had finally met some nice Germans." Women in urban areas like Berlin are often able to arrange delivery with the help of organizations that will set up services at a "trusted" hospital. These services are essentially donated, although various forms of copayment are often arranged. By law, the state is obligated to cover the costs for a hospital delivery. However, because the hospital's request for reimbursement is sent to the Social Welfare Office, which in turn is required to notify the Foreigner's Office, the patient risks the possibility of deportation. For these reasons, along with the amount of red tape involved, most hospitals prefer to skip this official process.

DOI: 10.4324/9781003307532-8

At the Migrant Clinic, the doctor typed up a referral letter to a lab that collaborates with them, printed it out, and handed it to Sarah with a set of directions. She then called up a hospital that provides two beds per month for undocumented women. Sarah was lucky; she was already eight months pregnant and her due date approaching fast, but there was still a bed available and a "reservation" was made for her. Many migrant women appear only in the third trimester, out of fear of their status being discovered, while others simply appear at a hospital when birth is imminent and pose as a tourist. Many undocumented women have circumstances that would cover the costs for care and delivery. For example, if they are refugees awaiting a decision on their asylum case, the state is obligated to cover the costs. If the father of the child is German or possesses insurance coverage, he is asked to contribute to the costs of the birth. In most cases, reimbursement can occur through the social welfare system or via his insurance, although it may be retroactive and dependent on submission of a birth certificate. For this reason, the physicians quizzed Sarah extensively about her situation.

Protecting the health of expectant mothers is a high priority in the German policy environment. The 1968 Maternity Protection Act codifies differential treatment of pregnant women, rationalized by protecting children's health, which includes limiting the activities of pregnant and nursing women, spelling out the conditions for maternity leave, and making it easier for women to combine working with childbearing. The Maternity Protection Act, or *Mutterschutzgesetz*, establishes a time frame six weeks before and eight weeks following birth, during which all women are accorded these protections. For an undocumented woman, this represents a crucial period during which she cannot be legally deported. Conceptualized as a humanitarian provision, migrant women are constructed as deserving of state protection while pregnant. This is a curious reversal of their experiences of deportability in everyday life, reflecting an apparent contradiction in German policy. Nonetheless, there are instances in which the *Mutterschutz* has not been honored by immigration authorities.

To formally take advantage of the *Mutterschutz*, the woman must register at the local courthouse and then apply for a residency permit at the Foreigner's Office. At that point, she will be given a *Duldung* (a temporary suspension of deportation), which authorizes access to prenatal care and covers delivery costs. If the woman does not register, her child is born into illegality and it becomes increasingly difficult to obtain a birth certificate, so that the child is at risk of becoming "undocumented" in the most literal sense of the word. Even without the registration and formal *Duldung*, pregnant women are entitled to the protection period. The formal paperwork makes compensation for costs related to the delivery possible, so that many hospitals encourage women to complete this step. However, by making themselves known to officials, they also draw the attention of the police, who will come looking for them once the *Mutterschutz* period is over. This fear is reinforced by actual and rumored instances where the policy was not honored by authorities. As a result, from the parents' perspective, the benefits of applying for a *Duldung* are limited and short term, whereas the price is visibility, state surveillance, and greater susceptibility to deportation. Staying "hidden" can provide considerably greater freedom. This calculation, combined with a generalized distrust of German authorities, leads many women to refuse to complete the process of formal application.

During her last trimester, Sarah became very lonely as she was mostly isolated without family or friends. Sarah called up Auntie Vinolia, an acquaintance and respected member of Berlin's West African community. Auntie Vinolia, who speaks impeccable German, joined Sarah for the remaining appointments and eventually even attended the birth. She also had the foresight to request a letter from the hospital for Sarah to carry on her person, so that when she went into labor, the ambulance would take her to that particular hospital and not simply the nearest one. This would ensure she would be taken to a safe place, free from suspicious hospital staff who might be inclined to call the police.

One morning, I rode the subway with Sarah and Auntie Vinolia following a meeting with the obstetrician and hospital social worker. The social worker had urged Sarah to apply for her *Duldung* at the Foreigner's Office as soon as possible. It would provide her a temporary legal status, some money and clothing for the baby, and ensure that the hospital would be compensated for the delivery. On the ride home, I asked Auntie Vinolia when they planned on going to apply, but she dismissed the idea. "No, she cannot go there. They will keep her passport and fingerprint her, and then they will want to deport her." When I reminded her about the rights Sarah had to certain benefits, Auntie Vinolia looked me straight in the eye and said, "We are Africans. We HAVE no rights" (Castañeda 2008).

This chapter discusses how migration policies are inscribed on bodies in ways that are gendered and gendering, in addition to intersecting with race and other factors (Castañeda 2008; Chavez 2004, 2017; Goldade 2009, 2011; Sargent 2006; Tober et al. 2006; Tormey 2007; Willen 2005). Women's experiences of migration, and their relationship to a host country, vary significantly from those of migrant men. In addition to exploring women's health concerns more broadly, this chapter examines how migrant reproduction highlights notions of citizenship and belonging in various host nations. Building on the concept of "stratified reproduction" (Colen 2009; Ginsburg & Rapp 1991, 1995), it explores how immigrants' experiences in host countries are linked to xenophobic fears of loss of a national identity, specific forms of "reconquest," or "demographic theft" (Chavez 2004; Castañeda 2008; Tormey 2007). These constructions create notions of deservingness with very real political and economic consequences for the health of migrants and their families. The key questions that this chapter answers include the following: In what ways are health and illness gendered and gendering for migrants? What unique issues come into play with reproduction, among all genders? How does a critical approach help us understand the impacts of gender on migrants' experiences of health? How does a critical examination of issues related to migrant sexuality help us understand the ways in which people contest and renegotiate the meanings behind citizenship and belonging? What issues do the experiences of lesbian, gay, bisexual, transgender, or otherwise-queer identifying (LGBTQ+) migrants highlight?

Critical Approaches to Understanding Gender, Sexuality, and Migrant Health

Gender is one of the fundamental social categories anchoring and shaping immigration patterns (Hondagneu-Sotelo 2003). A critical lens offers explicit attention to social, political, and economic power that is necessary to understand the interplay between gender, sexuality, and health. A feminist approach, in particular, helps decenter women away from tropes of victimhood, sexual behaviors, and reproduction as the primary loci of their migrant experiences and instead focus on their broader social relationships as well as creative networks of support.

The concept of *gendered geographies of power* helps explore migrant women's agency as constrained by time, space, and various layers of power inequalities (Pessar & Mahler 2003; Stock 2012). In many cases, women migrants experience greater social and economic mobility than in their home countries. However, their status gains are not universal, as some women face substantial exploitation, social isolation, and discrimination in the migration process and in receiving countries (Viruell-Fuentes & Schulz 2009).

Shifts in Family Structures, Conjugal Relationships, and Gender Roles

Scholars have examined how women's relations of kinship, care, and identity are impacted by migration patterns and policies, especially as this relates to transnational and mixed-status families living in environments shaped by deportability (Boehm 2012; Hondagneu-Sotelo 2001; Menjívar et al. 2016; Pessar & Mahler 2003; Segura & Zavella 2007). While less research has focused on family members who "stay behind" in sending communities, there is evidence that women in these situations often assume roles and responsibilities previously held by male partners, such as managing finances, and thus frequently experience increased autonomy, engage in new skills, and expand their social networks (Boehm 2012; Menjívar & Agadjanian 2007). Men who stay behind may have greater responsibility for children, often upending conventional understandings of gender roles in the family (Gallo 2006; Hoang & Yeoh 2011).

In addition, people form new partnerships and reconfigure existing forms of intimacy within families following migration, often leading to changing gender relations and practices (González-López 2005; Hirsch 2003; Walsh 2009). Partner or family separation may be part of a strategic long-term plan to benefit the entire household – for instance, through financial remittances or to enable other family members to pursue education or work (Mata-Codesal 2015; Pauli 2008). Research has uncovered both negative and positive effects of separation of spousal relationships as well as with extended family. Divorce, estrangement, and financial difficulties are often related to the difficulties of maintaining a transnational relationship, and these have broader consequences on well-being within households and communities. Several studies around the globe, for instance, have described the relationship between migration, infidelity, and increasing rates of HIV/AIDS in local communities (Agadjanian et al. 2011; Hirsch 2003; Padilla 2007; Smith & Yang 2005). On the other hand, transnational partnerships may be empowering, especially when couples are able to integrate separation into understandings of shared life projects, such as home building and upward social mobility (Gray 2011; Kwon 2015; Mata-Codesal 2015).

Marriage and family planning goals are frequently transformed and renegotiated in the context of migration. In one long-term study of sexuality and reproductive health among Mexican migrant women in the U.S., couples engaged in new ways of practicing intimacy that marked a clear shift from previous generations (Hirsch 2003), especially through intra-partner egalitarianism and mutual trust. However, in another study on fertility practices in the post-migration context with Roma women in Spain (Gamella 2018), shifting gender ideologies were strongly impacted by the involvement of extended family, education levels, and encounters with health care and social services.

The ways in which migration researchers have conceptualized families has shifted dramatically in the past decades, alongside broader developments in social science scholarship. This includes attention to intimate practices beyond "blood"-based kinship and traditional conceptualizations of biological family, as well as accounting for non-heteronormative configurations and experiences, including same-sex partnerships, single-parent households, and chosen families. A critical approach thus focuses on how migration policies interact with sexuality- and gender-based hierarchies (including those implied by conventional meanings of family) to marginalize and exclude individuals and relationships (Luibhéid 2002, 2008).

Gender and Reproduction

Fertility patterns and shifts in family planning associated with migration have a long history of study, which continue to be important from a critical perspective as conceptualizations and practices of sexuality and reproduction are shaped by social, economic, and historical contexts. In addition to other ways in which migration is gendered and gendering, women's experiences and their relationship to a host country may vary significantly from those of men simply because, for example, pregnancy is a possibility. Pregnancy is a precarious time especially for undocumented women because it heightens their visibility – and subsequent deportability – due to the need to interact with the health care system and various state offices, as Sarah's case at the start of this chapter illustrated. Parenthood necessitates additional financial resources, results in loss of work time, and may contribute to a lack of mobility, which may be important considerations for women employed in labor sectors such as home health care, cleaning, or other forms of domestic work.

The analytical notion of *stratified reproduction* conceptualizes reproductive health, fecundity, birth experiences, and child rearing as hierarchically arranged so that it is empowered for some but stigmatized for others, particularly marginalized groups (Colen 2009; Ginsburg & Rapp 1991). In examining constructions of Latina reproduction in the U.S., Chavez argues that media representations "produce fears about the population growth of Latinos in American society, which in turn positions them as a possible threat to the 'nation,' that is, the 'people' as conceived in demographic and racial terms" (2004: 173). Anthropologists have provided case studies from across the globe to demonstrate how regulations and population policies become inscribed on the bodies of migrant women. For instance, in a study of Malian migrants in Paris (Sargent 2006), explicitly antinatalist discourse coexists with otherwise pronatalist French policies on family size. Women considered to be authentically "French" are encouraged to have children, while medical practitioners implicitly and explicitly discouraged high fertility among migrant Malian women, dissuading them from having large families by pushing contraception.

In addition to racial stratification, constructs of nationhood and citizenship impact how migrant reproduction is perceived in a host country. In a study of Nicaraguan migrant women in Costa Rica (Goldade 2009), an increase in the number of births among Nicaraguan mothers was implicated in declining health care resources in the country. This led to reproductive stigma against them and anxieties regarding their reproductive capacity. Particular notions of national belonging influencing perceptions of migrant mothers was also evident in a study of pregnant undocumented women in Tel Aviv, Israel (Willen 2005, 2010), where the availability of reproductive and infant health services for them represented a surprising exception to the overall hostile environment for migrants in otherwise pronatalist Israel. Israel, like other countries that practice a descent-based system of citizenship called the *jus sanguinis* or "right of blood" model, has been reluctant to draw migrants into the body politic based on unique conceptualizations of citizenship and national belonging.

By contrast, many other nations, including the U.S. and France, follow a territorial or *jus soli* model, meaning that anyone born within the borders of the state is eligible for citizenship. The juridical model of citizenship in a host country has marked implications for migrant parents and their children. To highlight this, a study of pregnant Black women in Ireland (Tormey 2007) traced the transition from a *jus solis* to *jus sanguinis* model of citizenship. A Constitutional Amendment was proposed in 2004 amid anxieties over women arriving in Ireland on what is termed "maternity holiday," that is, to give birth and acquire Irish citizenship for their child. Specific ideas of morality were invoked to underscore rhetorics of exclusion, with foreign-born, non-citizen mothers considered to have "no real connection" to Ireland, and thus lacking in loyalty to the nation. This purported connection is ultimately one of bloodline; however, what it means to be "Irish" implicitly draws on ideas of race.

Attention to constructs of paternity is also required, as they are also flexible and inform particular notions of citizenship that are powerfully associated with rights and access to resources. Although anthropologists have analyzed migrant women's reproduction in several settings, less attention has focused on fatherhood and its relationship to constructs of the nation. In contrast to most nations of Western Europe and North America that follow a territorial model of citizenship, migrant children born in Germany do not automatically have the right to citizenship. This has led to unique practices regarding paternity and anxieties around what can be described as "demographic theft" (Castañeda 2008), which refers to a downward trend in native birth rates coupled with a simultaneous increase among foreigners. In the German case, legal loopholes designed to ensure the mother's autonomy have fostered an emergent market for false paternity claims. German men (or legal resident foreigners) can provide the means for undocumented women and their newborns to become regularized, although the extant of this practice is often exaggerated. The loopholes that allow such paternity claims further highlight the uneven social terrain of reproduction, because the very same law that empowers German mothers is perceived as suspect and dishonest when engaged by migrant women. As this example illustrates, the idea of "demographic theft" helps to illustrate the shift away from the *jus sanguinis* model of citizenship as well as juridico-cultural practices allowing for the separation of biological and social paternity.

Transnational Parenting

In addition to reproduction, scholarship has focused on transnational parenthood, or the physical separation of parents from their children and ways in which they form and maintain affective ties from a distance (Cordero 2021). As noted above, women's primary role as economic provider in the context of migration frequently shifts ideas of gender and mothering (Gamburd 2000; Parreñas 2001). Caretaking responsibilities may be taken up by grandmothers, husbands, siblings, or extended kin, although migrant mothers often remain involved in parenting and child rearing practices through, for example,regular communication and remittances. At the same time, structural inequalities play into these experiences, as legal status and social class strongly determine their ability to sustain long-distance familial ties, especially with their children (Carling et al. 2012; Lee 2021).

In other cases, children are born in the host country and, depending on the citizenship model in place, may become citizens there. This is linked the rise in mixed-status families in many countries, such as the U.S. (Castañeda 2019). Occasionally, children are born into literal "undocumentedness." Some parents may be reluctant to obtain a birth certificate for their children, or to submit a record of the birth to the municipality or to their country's embassy. Without a record of their identity, children may miss opportunities for health services, including immunizations, regular health checkups, and starting school. These experiences impact the healthy development of children, who in the worst cases may become "illegalized" or stateless themselves, without adequate legal protection from any country.

From an international rights perspective, children are generally viewed as requiring and deserving of special protection. However, this is not always the case for migrant children. For instance, in Norway, restrictive immigration policies have undermined the state's commitment to protecting children (Karlsen 2016). A state's interest in border control is often in direct tension with its obligations to protect children; this tension is frequently negotiated in encounters with health care service providers, in which frontline staff must often make difficult decisions – operating as gatekeepers on behalf of the state – to include or exclude children from services. Thus, despite discourse positioning children as particularly deserving of state protection, migrant children are frequently negatively impacted by the management and control of unwanted migration, especially through restrictions on access to welfare.

Migration and Masculinities

While the feminization of migration has been a topic of study as job opportunities for women have increased around the globe, shifting masculinities is another area of scholarship with implications for health. As women migrate to fill global demands for domestic service work, men find themselves increasingly managing households and childcare. This frequently reconfigures understandings of masculinity and parenthood (Gallo 2006; Hoang & Yeoh 2011). While transnational fatherhood has received far less attention than transnational motherhood, there is some evidence that fathers face more barriers in maintaining emotional and intimate ties with family members who remain behind, especially children (Fiałkowska 2019). On the other hand, separation from families often compels men to reevaluate their parenting roles and devise new strategies for maintaining close ties.

Deportation practices are particularly salient to the topic of gender and especially masculinity. Increased rates of deportation across the globe have led to "a gendered racial removal program" (Golash-Boza & Hondagneu-Sotelo 2013), as the masculinization of deportation (and "deportability" of male migrants) corresponds to the growing demand for low-skilled female labor. When they can no longer provide economically for their families, deportation may be experienced as emasculating. This may increase emotional detachment and lead to long-standing consequences for family cohesion (Fiałkowska 2019).

Sexual and Queer Migrations

Sexuality is an important area in which people contest and renegotiate the meanings behind citizenship and belonging (as well as "illegality," specifically), often intersecting with other shifting relations of power related to race, gender, class, and geopolitics (Luibhéid 2008). "Sexual migration" refers to mobilities that are directly or indirectly motivated by sexuality and may include

> transportation of practices across international borders, their lives in their places of origin, their exposure to local and foreign sexual ideologies prior to migrating, their agency in adapting and appropriating ideologies and

> practices prevalent in both home and host countries, and the transformations in sexual identities and behaviors
>
> *Carrillo 2004: 58*

that may occur after migration.

Studies of sexual and queer migrations are able to critique the normalization of heterosexual institutions and practices (Manalansan 2006). Indeed, opportunities for migration are frequently shaped by heteronormative reasoning, excluding in many cases possibilities for reunification or transnational marriage for same-sex couples or those who identify as LGBTQ+. Thus, sexuality emerges as an important object of study because of its constitutive role in the formation of citizenship and conceptualizations of the nation.

LGBTQ+-identifying migrants frequently experience health-related vulnerabilities rooted in social and political inequalities. They are more likely to lack health insurance and regular access to care, in addition to facing barriers to appropriate care and encountering stigma regarding their identity, sexual orientation, or gender expression in clinical spaces (Kline 2020). People who are both LGBTQ+-identifying and immigrants may experience overlapping forms of marginalization due to being a sexual and gender minority as well as a racial and ethnic minority. LGBTQ+ im/migrants with precarious immigration statuses (who may identify as "undocuqueer") are particularly susceptible to interlocking forms of oppression such as xenophobia, racism, and discrimination (Kline 2020).

Sexual Health

Research on migrants' sexual health is limited but has focused mainly on risks and accessibility issues, often without adequate recommendations for health promotion. This is another area where attention to structural factors is critical, with implications for changing organizational and societal factors linked to immigration and asylum systems. Overall, migrants appear to experience poor sexual and reproductive health outcomes, often due to the failure of policies to effectively reach them.

Legal status is, in fact, a key determinant of risk, as noted by one study on sexual health among refugees, asylum seekers, and undocumented migrants in Belgium and the Netherlands (Keygnaert et al. 2014). Both a lack of agency and sexual and reproductive health literacy have been shown to be critical components (Sime 2016). Often, this literacy is hampered by socioeconomic background, societal taboos, and the disruption to schooling because of displacement, leading to low levels of, for example, knowledge about contraceptive use. This, in turn, places people at greater risk for sexually transmitted infections and unintended pregnancy. For instance, a study of undocumented migrants in Japan found that there was a higher chance among migrants than the general population that their pregnancies were unwanted or unexpected (Calain-Watanabe & Lee 2012).

Intimate Partner Violence

Vulnerability to violence is shaped by structural factors, both at an individual and at a larger collective level through inequities in resources (including information) and barriers to service provision. Many migrants, because of stigma, discrimination, and access limitations, are marginalized and rendered invisible, increasing their risk of adverse sexual and reproductive health outcomes.

Structural violence often precipitates violence within households and intimate relationships (Alexander & Fernandez 2014), with numerous studies linking legal status and women's vulnerability to intimate partner violence (see Okeke-Ihejirika et al. 2020). In addition to arriving with limited support systems, they may struggle with shifting gender roles and changing family dynamics. Undocumented persons, especially women, are frequently disconnected from extended family and supportive social ties, and they may be financially dependent on abusive partners. This makes them less likely to seek out assistance in the case of intimate partner violence. Furthermore, in many host countries, services and policies are not well suited to immigrant women's needs and may even undermine their ability to seek out solutions. For example, an overview of intimate partner violence among immigrants in Canada (Okeke-Ihejirika et al. 2020) noted that studies tended to "pathologize" immigrant women and their wider communities in both overt and subtle ways by locating the causes and occurrences of intimate partner violence in their cultural backgrounds. Ideological "clashes" between traditional gender roles and Western values were seen as setting the stage for violence in domestic settings. However, especially from a critical perspective, it is important to account for the various forms of structural and institutional violence that instigate and reinforce intimate partner violence as individuals, families, and communities deal with displacement and dislocation. In addition to patriarchal ideologies and practices, people's vulnerability is mediated by the systemic violences they experience every day.

Young migrants, in particular, are at high risk of gender-based and sexual violence (Garin et al. 2016). However, intimate and sexual activity is frequently conceptualized as the realm of adults, even though young people are at increased risk for adverse sexual and reproductive health outcomes in crisis situations (Mason-Jones & Nicholson 2018). Children and youth are often further invisibilized when migration is considered the realm of adults and intact families, rather than an activity also undertaken by young people on their own. These biases frequently result in their unique needs being overlooked, as their marginalization and experiences of structural violence go unrecognized.

Conclusion

This chapter examined how migration is gendered and gendering, with specific implications for health. Alongside sexuality, these experiences overlap with race and conceptualizations of national belonging. Ideas about reproduction, in particular, have important implications for conceptualization of migrant deservingness and access to services. As we have seen, a critical approach is important because structural and institutional conditions impact experiences of sexuality, reproduction, family, parenting, and intimate relationships, often deleteriously, because of migration, displacement, and separation.

The next chapter examines the violences associated with immigration enforcement, detention, and deportation and their impact on health. Using a critical perspective, it lays out how enforcement policies and their subsequent actions perpetuate health disparities, exacerbate existing health-related vulnerabilities related to legal status, and in addition to creating new health concerns, threatening the health and well-being of entire communities. Assessing the complex relationship between immigration enforcement and health requires adopting critical theoretical perspectives that emphasize systemic factors and the connection between social phenomena and political processes that influence poor health.

9

HEALTH IMPACTS OF ENFORCEMENT, DETENTION, AND DEPORTATION

Along the U.S./Mexico border, undocumented parents face an excruciating choice. If their children need specialty medical treatment in another city, they must weigh this with potential risk of their deportation. In addition to the dangers associated with daily encounters with immigration authorities, a series of permanent checkpoints create a sense of regional confinement, which affects the lives of all residents, regardless of whether they are citizens or migrants, whether they are recent arrivals or have lived in the U.S. for decades. These checkpoints are located up to 100 miles from the border along all major highways that lead into the interior of the U.S. and are staffed 24 hours a day, seven days a week, forcing travelers to pass through one if they travel to the interior.

Eight-year-old Sofia was recently diagnosed with leukemia. The only treatment available for her complex pediatric case was at MD Anderson Cancer Center in Houston, which lies on the other side of the immigration checkpoints on U.S. Highway 281. Although Sofia was a U.S. citizen and her medical care was covered through Medicaid, a public insurance, her mother was undocumented. This meant that she would not be allowed to accompany Sofia to the hospital, even though she is her parent. Even a copy of her medical records – accompanied by a letter from her physician addressed to U.S. Border Patrol and Customs – was not likely to suffice in allowing her mother to cross into the interior of the state. There was simply no guarantee that she wouldn't be deported if she approached the immigration checkpoint with her child.

In disbelief and anguish, the physician treating Sofia told me, "She had to put her daughter on a Greyhound bus, with her 14-year-old brother as the guardian," accompanying her on the trip to Houston. He added,

DOI: 10.4324/9781003307532-9

> It's just immoral for us as a society to expect a mother to stay behind while her 8-year-old daughter has to travel 400 miles away for cancer treatment. To tell her, "No, you're not allowed to go." In what world is that alright?
>
> *Physician cited in Castañeda 2019*

Indeed, migrants who are unauthorized or have unclear legal status are under constant threat of being detained or deported. This example highlights the role of interior immigration enforcement practices that limit access to medical care far from the physical border itself. Inspection and policing practices have expanded both within and beyond territorial boundaries, making life increasingly uncertain for immigrants in interior communities. In the U.S., this situation worsened after authorities clamped down on approving temporary authorization for travel for humanitarian reasons. In the past, border patrol agents were more likely to exercise discretion in deciding not to detain or deport parents with sick children or other extenuating circumstances.

This case also illustrates how it is not just undocumented people who are affected but also their family members – including family members who are U.S. citizens, such as Sofia. In the case of mixed-status families – that is, families that contain varied constellations of citizens, permanent legal residents, undocumented immigrants, and individuals in legal limbo – immigration enforcement practices have broad spillover effects on others living in the same household, leading to a form of multigenerational punishment (Enriquez 2015).

Immigration enforcement policies and activities produce detrimental effects on migrant adults and children, as well as larger social units such as families, neighborhoods, and entire communities. A significant body of research has examined the direct and indirect effects of immigration policy and law enforcement on well-being. As this chapter illustrates, everyday life with a pervasive fear of deportation negatively impacts psychological, physical, and emotional health. Aggressive immigration regimes impact a variety of health behaviors and encourage racism and discrimination, creating additional stressors. Living with constant surveillance transforms public spaces into environments of risk, resulting in some people excluding themselves from health-promoting activities, places, and resources. Thus, this chapter examines how enforcement policies and their subsequent actions – arrest, detention, and deportation – perpetuate health disparities, exacerbate existing vulnerabilities related to status, and create new health problems (Boehm 2016; De León 2015; Duncan 2014; Kline & Castañeda 2019; Lopez et al. 2017). These experiences are highly gendered, with enforcement usually targeting men more prominently than women (Brotherton & Barrios 2011; Golash-Boza & Hondagneu-Sotelo 2013; Kohli et al. 2011). The detrimental impact of deportation and detention disrupts family relationships and produces emotional, economic, and psychosocial stressors, and children whose parents have been deported experience a host of social concerns and mental health problems. While the U.S. context provides one of the best examples of how these oppressive processes work, and is thus somewhat overrepresented in this chapter, other global cases are included as well. The key questions that this chapter answers include the following: What are the health impacts of living under a "deportation regime"? What is the added effect of interior policing? What are the impacts of enhanced immigration enforcement, such as interior policing and raids, on immigrant health? What are the effects on health of communities? Does regularization/legalization lead to improvements in health?

Critical Approaches to Understanding Health Impacts of Enforcement, Detention, and Deportation

Assessing the complex relationship between immigration enforcement and health requires adopting critical perspectives that emphasize systemic factors and the connection between social phenomena and political processes that influence poor health (Leischow & Milstein 2006; Luke & Stamatakis 2012). Securitization discourse and practices have dominated migration management since the 1990s, relying on dual processes of externalization (i.e., outsourcing extraterritorial activities to sending and transit countries) as well as the internalization of border controls, as the opening vignette to this chapter illustrates. These "deportation regimes" criminalize unauthorized migration and seek to control mobility by employing a range of national/federal, state/provincial, and local resources (De Genova & Peutz 2010; Dowling & Inda 2013). This has expanded migration management beyond the physical international border and toward the interior of nations, accompanied by the proliferation of inspection checkpoints, surveillance technologies, and detention practices.

The fiercely punitive positions toward immigrants that dominate in many nations today draw on other forms of exclusion by race and social class (Garcia 2017; Stumpf 2006). Beginning at the turn of the 21st century and intensifying since, immigration enforcement in many nations began to function by fusing together criminal and immigration law. *Crimmigration* – the nexus of immigration policy and policing that emerged over the past 30 years, most evident in the U.S. – refers to the intersecton of criminal law and immigration law, the merger of which produces complex legal and practical challenges (García Hernández 2015).

In some settings, rather than devolution to the local level, deportations are outsourced to third countries. For example, "assistance programs" arranged by the EU often provide the mechanisms for mass expulsions to occur in North Africa, rather than from Europe. Malian migrants, for example, are sent to and then deported from Algeria to reception centers in Niger as part of EU-funded return and reintegration programs (Sylla & Cold-Ravnkilde 2021).

In the U.S., immigration enforcement has shifted to local levels (e.g., states, counties, municipalities) (Fix & Tumlin 1997; Suárez-Orozco & Suárez-Orozco 2009). As a result, immigrant communities experience heightened chances of encountering police and profiling practices. Initiatives like 287(g), Secure Communities (S-Comm), and the Priority Enforcement Program (PEP) encourage coordination between local law enforcement agencies and ICE. This means that with any traffic stop, undocumented drivers risk detention and deportation. While such programs purportedly intend to target migrants with violent criminal convictions, evidence shows that half of those deported via Secure Communities, for instance, had either no criminal conviction or a minor one, such as a traffic offense (Kohli et al. 2011). Along with these approaches comes an assumption that people will "self-deport" if access to social services, including health care, is removed. It assumes that even without concerted effort to impact lives through heightened enforcement, people would be convinced to leave the country rather than stay in a hostile environment.

However, "aggressive complicity" between local and federal authorities "produces a widespread and intense feeling of deportability among individuals throughout the wider community" (Alexander & Fernandez 2014: 16). These efforts have not been without pushback, as enforcing federal immigration law distracts local authorities from their primary duties, in addition to fostering fear in communities. Distrust in institutions impacts public safety and security, making people less likely to participate as active members of their communities and making them hesistant to report crimes, even when they are victims. This lack of engagement in civic life impacts overall population health (Asch et al. 1998; Carpiano 2006; Davis & Henderson 2003; Lysakowski et al. 2016; Subramanian et al. 2002). Although actual levels of risk to detention and deportation vary widely, both prior experiences and rumors circulate in communities and become internalized by individuals. This *deportability* thus becomes a powerful presence in the daily lives of migrants, even for those who are not undocumented themselves (De Genova 2002; Quesada et al. 2011; Talavera et al. 2010). In response, migrants may delay treatment of illness or forgo health care altogether.

Pathogenic law enforcement (Bourgois & Schonberg 2009) or *pathogenic policing* (Kline 2019) refers to the ways in which enforcement activities destabilize the lives of migrants (and other marginalized groups) in ways that produce negative effects on health. This concept has analytic utility in understanding the disproportionate health risks and unequal health outcomes that migrants face. *Socioecological models* can further illuminate the various levels – those of the individual, of social relationship, of community and broad societal factors – that shape the everyday health impacts of immigration status.

The stress and mental anguish of poverty, racialization, racism, and discrimination are experienced intersubjectively and can be productively thought about as *familial vulnerability*, a theoretical concept that broadly accounts for how the structural vulnerability of any individual family member can have a deleterious impact on other members (Logan et al. 2021). Finally, drawing on the public health concept of the "illness pyramid," a *deportation pyramid* can be used to describe vulnerability for migrant families and others in the community (Dreby 2012). In this model, the top of the pyramid is reserved for those directly affected when they are detained or deported; lower levels highlight the indirect impacts that trickle downward to affect children (including those who are citizens), to the classmates and teachers of those children, to legal immigrants whose stability also feels threatened, to others in the community – such as citizen neighbors – who would not seem to be affected but actually are as well.

Fear of Deportation and Effects on Mental and Emotional Health

Life in illegality and the constant threat of deportation – either one's own deportability or that of family members – disrupts people's sense of security. Anti-immigrant rhetoric, laws, policies, and enforcement activities produce fear and anxiety in communities (Alexander & Fernandez 2014; Brabeck & Xu 2010; Dreby 2012; Hagan et al. 2011; Menjívar 2011; Talavera et al. 2010). Undocumented immigrants and their family members experience a pervasive fear of deportation that negatively impacts their psychological, emotional, and physical health (Cavazos-Rehg et al. 2007; Hacker et al. 2011; Hacker et al. 2012; Sullivan & Rehm 2005).

Even the threat of deportation can provoke poor health. Research has documented significant associations between worry about deportation and depression and anxiety (Valdez et al. 2013; Yoshikawa & Kalil 2011). One study found that a full 68% of Latino respondents – regardless of their own legal status – worried that they, a family member, or a close friend might be deported (Lopez & Minushkin 2008). Furthermore, psychological and financial consequences of detention and deportation affect family members living in the country of origin, who also experience anxiety and panic when losing contact with their family member, or prolonged periods without information about their whereabouts or well-being (Brabeck et al. 2011).

Thus, regardless of their own legal status, immigrants may report higher levels of stress due to deportation fear, which impacts their overall mental and emotional well-being (Hacker et al. 2011). They are significantly more likely to experience challenges in employment, physical health problems, psychological distress, and acculturative stress (Arbona et al. 2010; Cavazos-Rehg et al. 2007; Hacker et al. 2011). Hostile policy environments result in intense feelings of anxiety and depression (Cavazos-Rehg et al. 2007; Dreby 2012; Williams 2003). Some turn to self-medicating with alcohol and other drugs. Others simply suffer, as there are no mental health services available to them, or they may no longer maintain friendships outside the home, remaining socially isolated. In a study of Haitian immigrants' mental health in the Dominican Republic (Kaiser et al. 2015), individuals' experiences with prior detention or deportation, or knowing someone who had had these experiences, were associated with higher anxiety symptomology. Participants reported feeling like "little toys," due to the potential for arbitrary arrests in their everyday lives.

Physical Health Impacts of Deportability

While the distinction between mental/emotional health and physical conditions is at its core an artificial one, it is important to consider specifically how chronic fear can aggravate some health conditions and create risks for others. Fear of deportation has been associated with poorer self-perceived health (Cavazos-Rehg et al. 2007) and has been shown to exacerbate pre-existing physical conditions such as high blood pressure and diabetes (Cavazos-Rehg et al. 2007; Salas et al. 2013). In one U.S.-based study, fear of deportation exacerbated depression, high blood pressure, and anxiety and left migrants with a range of physical symptoms including headaches and hair loss (Hacker et al. 2011). The association between worry about deportation and cardiovascular risk factors has been empirically studied (in addition to self-reported outcomes) using reference points such as BMI, waist circumference, and continuous measures of systolic and pulse pressure (Torres et al. 2018). This further underscores the spillover effects beyond the individual, adding to the literature on the health impacts of deportation worry by illustrating how it activates the stress response system, including faster heart rate, inflammation, and heightened immune response.

Effects on Health Service Access and Health-Seeking Behavior

Another important issue is avoidance of or decreased access to medical services, as evidenced by lower rates of utilization (Heyman et al. 2009; Maldonado et al. 2013; Rhodes et al. 2015). Policies such as enhanced documentation requirements or the presence of police or border patrol agents in the vicinity of health facilities creates worry, and several studies have described the connection between local law enforcement activity and health care access (Asch et al. 1995, 1998; Berk & Schur 2001; Castañeda 2009; Magalhaes et al. 2010; McGuire & Georges 2003).

In addition, with increased police presence, immigrants are more susceptible to discrimination and racial profiling (Menjívar 2011), more likely to avoid public spaces (including government organizations and NGOs, schools, and places of worship) (Menjivar 2011), and be less willing to report a crime (Hacker et al. 2011). Even though medical facilities – like schools and places of worship – are generally considered "sensitive locations," where immigration raids ought not to occur, fear of deportation still keeps some people away, leading to delayed or deferred care with potentially significant public health implications for all. At the same time, health care systems, like schools and other institutions, often develop their own policies to accommodate migrant populations.

As part of the condition of deportability, people's hesitation is due in equal part to unsubstantiated rumors and actual enforcement events that have occurred in their community. For instance, there may be anecdotes about Border Patrol agents or vehicles waiting outside of hospitals. How often the fear of deportation translates into people forgoing care remains unclear and difficult to measure; presumably, it leads to more severe health issues and more costly emergency department visits.

Immigration Raids

The emotional, psychological, and material tolls of interior policing efforts on individuals and families is devastating and well documented (Capps et al. 2007; Dowling & Inda 2013; Kline & Castañeda 2019). One uniquely distressing practice with emerging evidence of severe health impacts is the home raid, in which agents enter a residence, often in the predawn hours when occupants are asleep. Seeking to detain undocumented immigrants, they often appear in body armor and with guns drawn, surrounding the residence, and pounding on doors. Often, additional persons suspected of having an unauthorized legal status may be detained as "collateral" arrests, a process rooted in racial profiling (Lopez et al. 2017). Children are frequently witnesses to these activities. Another common practice is workplace raids. In these cases, children may return home from school at the end of the day and find no parents in the home.

Scholars studying the health implications of immigration raids have found that the presence of such activities led to higher levels of stress and lower self-related health scores and other negative health impacts in communities in which raids occur (Lopez et al. 2017). Even rumors of immigration raids can lead to high levels of anxiety in a community. People report feeling more restricted in their movements, limiting their activities and social networks, and less able to use services following immigration raids, reflecting a reduction in control and negatively affecting social capital (Cavazos-Rehg et al. 2007).

Health Issues during the Detention or Deportation Process

Detention itself negatively impacts health and human dignity. In addition to its traumatizing effects, detained individuals may experience various forms of mistreatment, a lack of due process for reporting violations of their rights, and inadequate access to health care. Among detained Salvadoran deportees in the U.S., for instance, 20% reported the use of force during arrest (e.g., shoving, throwing to the ground; most of these involved excessive force), and 31% were denied access to adequate food and water while held in detention facilities (Phillips et al. 2006). A study of female detainees in Arizona noted inadequate access to mental/emotional health care as well as prenatal care (Rabin 2009).

By its very nature, detention involves uncertainty about length of time and anticipation of long-term family separation (Brabeck et al. 2014). These contribute to experiences of psychological distress, including frustration, anger, despondency, and suicidality (Keller et al. 2003). These experiences worsen with increased length of detention and are generally not countered by mental health services, which are frequently lacking in detention centers. For family members left behind, the palpable absence of a loved one results in additional health consequences. For people who have experienced state-sponsored kidnapping and murders in their countries of origin, the sudden "disappearance" of a family member can be particularly traumatic (Brabeck et al. 2011).

LGBTQ+ individuals face unique dangers in the detention process (Tabak & Levitan 2014). They may experience sexual assault, harassment, or violence, particularly if singled out for their perceived non-conformity with heterosexual gender norms. These experiences have the potential to exacerbate other mental or emotional stressors, leading to increases in anxiety and depression. Furthermore, medical care in detention centers may be inadequate or inappropriate for LGBTQ+ individuals, who suffer unique challenges regarding care appropriate to their needs, including hormone therapy or HIV treatment. Each of these experiences is compounded in the context of detention by frequent and severe stigmatization, isolation, and even solitary confinement (Furman et al. 2016).

The process of arrest and detention of children has particularly worrisome physical and mental health consequences. This includes a lack of protection of children's basic rights, with reports noting maltreatment by officials, including failure to notify Child Protective Services when necessary, the denial of access to legal representation and to respective home country consulates, being held for unreasonable periods of time, and/or being held in unsafe conditions (Benjet et al. 2009).

Impacts of Deportation on Children

Through spillover effects, a parent's legal vulnerability can affect children and influence their development (Suárez-Orozco et al. 2011; Yoshikawa & Kalil 2011). At different levels, children experience a variety of risk factors linked to parental vulnerability to deportation, including psychological distress, economic insecurity linked to parents' work conditions, and housing instability. However, they may also benefit from a range of protective factors, such as supportive family interactions, that may be able to buffer adverse effects.

Several concepts are useful here to complement structural approaches when understanding the effects of family separation on children. For instance, *attachment theory* suggests that a strong relationship with a caregiver is critical to children's sense of security, and is fundamental to learning developmental, emotional, and social regulation skills that are required throughout the life course (Bowlby & Ainsworth 2013). *Ambiguous loss* clarifies developmental implications when parents are physically absent but still psychologically present as part of a child's life (Boss 2006). The ambiguity produced by this situation may cause children to internalize stress and develop symptoms such as anxiety or depression. Insights from these perspectives have been useful in understanding the experiences of children whose parents are incarcerated and can be extended to migrant families who have faced detention or deportation. *Adverse childhood events* – such as family separation – refer to disruptions that affect healthy development and put children at risk for future illness. These accumulate over the life course and are associated with increased likelihood of cardiovascular disease and suicide, in addition to broader social impacts such as unemployment (Miranda & Legha 2019). *Toxic stress* is a concept that considers the result of repetitive, prolonged, or intense adversity, which produces shifts in the production of stress hormones as the body remains at high alert. Importantly, strategic interventions can offset the impacts of such trauma. The *cumulative risk* perspective (Rutter 1979) argues that adverse effects from an event are more likely to result in the context of multiple risks over the life course. For instance, the health impacts following a parent's deportation is critically heightened when children have other risk factors present, such as poverty, discrimination, or instable housing arrangements. Adverse experiences resulting from such cumulative risk factors can result in severe biological and psychological changes in developing children (Shonkoff et al. 2009).

Some forms of family separation during the migration process involve voluntary decisions (which are nonetheless often forced by often dire economic circumstances) that may bring with them economic and social benefits despite the emotional costs. However, forced separations due to deportation incur all the emotional cost without any of the economic or social benefit. In a study on the intimate experiences of undocumented families in Brussels, the authors note that the state draws on "normative imaginaries" about the family, largely reflected in ideas of what makes a "good" parent and relying on universalized notions of childhood as "innocent" and stable, that is, largely free from the major disruptions caused by migration. These normative logics are then enacted to legitimize and designate undocumented families as "deportable," as "'illegality' is transposed … towards the private sphere of parenthood, framing the hardships suffered by these families as the mere result of 'bad' parenting (e.g. 'choosing' to raise their children in 'illegality')" (van Osch 2021: 14–15).

Deportations produce multiple traumas for children who may witness the arrest of a parent, then abruptly lose them as a caregiver along with a familiar home environment (McLeigh 2010). While all undocumented parents are at risk of involuntary separation from their families, on average more men than women are detained or deported (Golash-Boza & Hondagneu-Sotelo 2013). Children who remain must adapt to abrupt changes in household structure, often living with their newly single mothers or other relatives and facing great economic insecurity. The involuntary separation of parents and children creates economic and emotional hardship, while restrictive immigration policies may lead to resentment among children even post-reunification (Dreby 2015). Out of fear of having their children permanently removed from their custody, some parents are reluctant to disclose that they even have children (Capps et al. 2007), creating additional challenges to ensuring that they are receiving adequate care.

Scholars have begun to systematically measure the health consequences of parental deportation on children (Brabeck & Xu 2010; Chaudry et al. 2010; Delva et al. 2013; Gonzales 2011). The physical separation of parent and child, especially if it is abrupt, unsettles feelings of security. The overwhelming consensus is that parental deportation causes increased emotional and behavioral distress among children, including sleep problems, depression, anxiety, and problems in school (Baum 2010; Brabeck & Xu 2010; Capps et al. 2007; Chaudry et al. 2010; Dreby 2012). Children may internalize symptoms (depression, anxiety) or exhibit externalizing behaviors (withdrawal, aggression) (Makariev & Shaver 2010; Allen et al. 2015).

Those whose parents have been deported or detained are more likely to experience a host of social and mental health problems, including decreased school performance, depression, anxiety, and aggression and conduct issues (Allen et al. 2015; Brabeck et al. 2014; Suárez-Orozco et al. 2002,). The most common short-term psychological effects on children's health may include loss of appetite and sleeping changes (including nightmares), crying, feeling afraid, along with anxiety, withdrawal, anger–aggression, and clinginess (Chaudry et al. 2010). Some children also display developmental difficulties (e.g., speech delay) and behavioral and academic problems in school.

Family separations through deportation can thus be recognized as a form of "legal violence," affecting the well-being of children (Menjívar & Abrego 2012). In addition to actual separation, frequently worrying about family separation impacts children, who may exhibit high levels of stress, which may lead to poor mental health (Horner et al. 2014). Separating children from their parents, or the threat thereof, represents an adverse childhood event. This can cause irreparable harm through toxic stress, and prolonged exposure to highly stressful situations affects children's short- and long-term health. During abrupt separation, children may experience a flood of stress hormones (e.g., cortisol) washing over the brain and the body; while important for navigating short-term stress, if hyperactive for a prolonged period of time these hormones can increase the risk of complications like heart disease, diabetes, and even some forms of cancer. Furthermore, multiple traumas early in life can lead to post-traumatic stress disorder (PTSD) and other mental health issues later in life.

Impacts of Deportation on the Larger Family Unit

The economic consequences of deportation have enormous implications for the well-being of the larger household. Loss of income leads to economic hardships, such as problems paying bills, increasing debts, housing instability, food insecurity, and an inability to send remittances to families in origin countries (Chaudry et al. 2010). This insecurity quickly leads to crisis especially in families who have not yet paid off debts related to the migration process (Brabeck et al. 2011; Menjívar & Abrego 2012).

Deportation also creates changes in family structure and stability. In some cases, the loss of income and emotional support, coupled with housing instability and increased mental distress, can lead to family dissolution altogether. One study in the U.S. (Dreby 2012) found that one-quarter of families that experienced deportation were unable to keep their transnational family together. Despite changing trends over time, the overwhelming number of deportees continue to be male (Brotherton & Barrios 2011; Kohli et al. 2011), and newly single mothers are frequently under enormous economic stress without any resources to weather the conditions (Dreby 2012). For households that remain without a primary breadwinner because of deportation, precarious housing, food insecurity, psychological distress, and poverty are often inevitable. Shifts in childcare are often another result, as older siblings may need to step in and care for younger brothers and sisters (Dreby 2012).

As noted above, many women who experience the deportation of a male partner may be abruptly required to take on the household as a single parent. Sometimes this requires working multiple jobs or resorting to public assistance to meet the daily demands of rent, food, transportation, and childcare (Dreby 2015). Family structures may be further disrupted if children are relegated to foster care after their parents have been detained. This most heavy-handed form of state intervention into the intimate lives of families can sometimes even result in the loss of parental rights to their own children. The U.S. foster care system, for instance, is frequently entangled with structural prejudice against immigrant families (Rodriguez 2017). Parental deportation can translate into child abandonment by the legal system, even with no prior history or evidence of abuse or neglect, which can even lead to the termination of parental rights.

Impacts of Deportation on Communities

Raids and deportations have an afterlife. The consequences associated with heightened anti-immigrant policy environments reach beyond undocumented persons themselves, impacting others in their community (Androff et al. 2011; Cavazos-Rehg et al. 2007; Gonzales et al. 2013; Salas et al. 2013; Vargas & Ybarra 2016). Deportability exerts influence over the sense of security of entire neighborhoods by instilling fear and distrust of authorities, including local police, health professionals, social service professionals, and school staff (Dreby 2012; Menjívar & Abrego 2012). As a result of enforcement activities in neighborhoods, people may become less willing to drive, call an ambulance (Lopez et al. 2017), or call the police, even when they are victims or witnesses to a crime (Hacker et al. 2011; Sládková et al. 2012). Another result is that children of unauthorized parents may be kept out of school (Androff et al. 2011; Capps et al. 2007).

This disrupted sense of security reaches far beyond the undocumented population, extending to legal immigrants and even citizens who learn to be suspicious of authorities, fear family separation, experience discrimination, and may feel reduced optimism about their status in society (Becerra et al. 2013). Growing up in a climate of fear and distrust impacts a child's civic relationship to the government and authorities more generally, and they may perceive police as a threat instead of as a resource.

After Deportation: Return to Country of Origin

On return to their home country, deportees frequently face a stigmatized existence. They may be viewed as criminals or as failures, leading to them feeling demoralized (Brabeck et al. 2014). Research indicates that some of the long-term impacts include unemployment (Brotherton & Barrios 2011), frequent drug use, and reduced uptake of medical services and treatment (Brouwer et al. 2009). Women who are deported face higher risk for physical and sexual assault and are more likely to enter sex work due to financial need (Robertson et al. 2012).

Migrant parents who are deported, depending on national context, resources, and legal framework, may face the difficult decision of whether or not to take their children with them. If they place them in the care of others – the other parent, extended family members, or friends – children may experience less disruption but lack their parents' nurturing presence (Zayas 2010). Placement with relatives may be hindered by legal requirements. If parents leave their children behind with others, they face possibility that parental bonds may be severed, either because they lose the emotional connection or because child protective laws declare them to be "absent." As noted above, parental deportation can become translated into child abandonment by the legal system, even with no history or evidence of abuse or neglect. Instead, neglect becomes constituted by parental disappearance following detention or deportation and can even lead to the termination of parental rights – and ultimately even to the adoption of the child to another family – if parents are not given access or resources to participate in family reunification processes (Rodriguez 2017). For children who stay behind with a single parent, other impacts on their well-being may emerge, most notably economic insecurity.

On the other hand, if children join their parents, they face a move to a foreign country where they may not know the language or culture. Parental deportation thus may prompt the "de facto deportation" of children, even if they are citizens (Golash-Boza & Hondagneu-Sotelo 2013). On returning to their parents' home country, they are likely to lose access to any benefits they may hold as citizens, such as rights to education or health care (Brabeck et al. 2011; Dreby 2012; Lykes et al. 2013). They may find themselves in environments of extreme poverty and face severe economic insecurity in their households. They may not feel connected or that they belong and may experience discrimination (Boehm 2011). Finally, their education may be impacted as transitioning to a new school system may be challenging; sometimes transcripts or curricula are not recognized, and they may not read and write in the new language. All these experiences can result in lower educational and vocational readiness, in addition to impacting emotional and mental health (Zayas 2010).

Conclusion

As this chapter has illustrated, there are a number of health impacts casued by living under a deportation regime that shapes everyday life with the pervasive fear of surveillance, detention, and deportation, including enhanced immigration enforcement practices such as interior policing and raids. These intersect with vulnerabilities associated with poverty, racialization, and discrimination. Through spillover effects, parents' legal status can impact children's well-being, and deportation produces multiple health consequences beyond the individual, affecting other family members and communities at large. A critical perspective highlights how enforcement policies and their subsequent actions – arrest, detention, and deportation – perpetuate health disparities, exacerbate existing vulnerabilities related to status, and create new health problems.

The final topical chapter of the book, Chapter 10, brings us back to describe the unique circumstances of refugees and asylum seekers. Their experiences, while reflected throughout the book, also share some unique features that are worth examining in more detail. Their migrations frequently inspire a different moral response in host communities than other kinds of migrants, which opens some specific opportunities (e.g., legal status, more available access to health care) but also may bring with it overall poorer health outcomes and a more intimate surveillance by governments. This chapter uses a critical perspective to explore the complex relationship between governments and health care regimes, illness origins and treatments within refugee populations, and claims of legitimacy.

10

FORCED DISPLACEMENT

Refugee and Asylum Seeker Health

Talk of a "crisis" was already well underway when I volunteered in a reception center for asylum seekers in Giessen, a city in the central German state of Hessen in the summer of 2014. Over the past year, there had been a five-fold increase in people arriving, with the city of 80,000 taking on 21,000 temporary refugee residents as they were processed and awaited resettlement. At that time, the mood was still upbeat, and the local population was eager to help. People welcomed the newcomers, and the reception center was overwhelmed with donations of clothing and toys. Medical professionals volunteered their time. Despite this outpouring of support, the director of the reception center told me, "We are in a state of emergency." The numbers grew exponentially by the following year.

A decommissioned U.S. military base was used to house many of the refugees. The compound had a complicated history as a site of refuge: after World War II, it held ethnic Germans expelled from territories annexed by Poland and the Soviet Union; later it served as emergency reception center for refugees from the former East Germany. During the civil wars in the Balkans in the 1990s, asylum seekers came from Bosnia and Kosovo. Even back then, people filled the space past its capacity. Now people arrived from Syria, Afghanistan, Eritrea, Iraq, Iran, and Somalia, many haven taken a route across the western Balkans, traversing Turkey and Greece. Those who arrived had often journeyed for months, and most were exhausted and traumatized. At peak times, 5,000 were housed at once, and as space ran out, tent cities were erected. Most refugees stayed for a month, but some stayed up to three months, until they were informed about their resettlement destinations.

At the reception center, people were processed, housed, and provided with medical attention. The focus was primarily on vaccine-preventable diseases and gastrointestinal complaints. Vaccines were provided to all who needed them, especially following reports of polio outbreaks in Syria as well as mumps and chicken pox outbreaks in reception centers in Germany. Many had traveled for months under

DOI: 10.4324/9781003307532-10

conditions of poor hygiene, had been sleeping outside, and were vulnerable to various infections. Scabies and lice were prevalent. These preventable conditions reflected conditions of overcrowding, both during the journey and in the reception centers. Gastrointestinal complaints, usually linked to noroviruses and rotaviruses, also emerged but disappeared as quickly as hygienic conditions improved. On the way to Europe, people also encountered violence, huge fluctuations in climate, hunger, and thirst.

The director of the center emphasized to me that the medical condition of the refugees was "remarkably good," given what they had endured. Data underscored that the illnesses that they presented with in the reception centers were mostly acquired in Germany, not brought in from their homelands. Overall, the asylum seekers tended to have the same ailments as the local German population, in addition to those brought on by overcrowding. One exception were symptoms of depression, fear, dissociation, suicidality, and PTSD, which were identified in the medical clinic on site, but often had long-term effects as there remains a lack of specialists to deal with sequalae of torture, trauma, and displacement.

As the mood in the local population began to change with more asylum seekers arriving and longer stays in the already overcrowded centers, physicians and center administrators took to the media to explain that there was no health threat to the general population. One physician explained, "It's the refugees who are the vulnerable population, they are not dangerous." Nonetheless, fear of communicable disease was used to stoke anger, fear, and xenophobia among some segments of the local population.

Although their experiences have been woven throughout this book, refugees and asylum seekers represent distinct migrant groups that face unique health challenges and prospects (Banke-Thomas et al. 2019; Clarke et al. 2021). They frequently inspire a different moral response in host communities and may be viewed as more (or less) "deserving" than other kinds of migrants. While this opens some potential privileges, it still does not inoculate them from discrimination, various obstacles to well-being, and overall poorer health outcomes. While refugees and asylum seekers may have access to more state-sponsored services and welfare programs than, for example, undocumented migrants fleeing less visible or less recognized forms of violence, the barriers to adequate care are still numerous. Even when resettled after an extensive vetting process, negative public perceptions of refugees persist, with assumptions about their taking advantage of social services, along with their conflation with other immigrants as a single, homogeneous group (Lawler and Tolley 2017). Unique to asylum seekers and refugees is their intimate contact with state governments, in both their home countries in the form of political violence and in the receiving countries that decide which persons are "real" applicants through extensive processes of examination. This chapter examines the complex relationship between state governments and health care regimes, illness origins and treatments within refugee populations, and claims of legitimacy (Fassin & D'Halluin 2005; Ticktin 2011). Key questions that this chapter answers include the following: What are some obstacles to health and well-being for refugees and asylum seekers from a structural perspective? What are the different approaches to understanding mental and emotional health issues in this population? How do claims of legitimacy affect health care seeking behaviors? What are some uniquely gendered experiences for refugees? What is resilience and what are the ways refugees operationalize this to aid in their situation?

Critical Approaches to Understanding Forced Displacement: Refugee and Asylum Seeker Health

A refugee is defined as a person who has been forced to flee their country of origin and is unable or unwilling to return because of a well-founded fear of being persecuted because of their race, religion, nationality, membership of a particular social group, or political opinion. The 1951 Geneva Convention is the primary international instrument of refugee law, defining who is a refugee and the kind of legal protection, assistance, and social rights they may receive from signatory countries. It was initially designed with a focus on European refugees in the aftermath of World War II; however, a revision, the 1967 Protocol, expanded the scope of the Convention as the problem of displacement grew globally.

An asylum seeker is a person seeking international protection, who has applied to a specific country for sanctuary but whose case is still in process. Thus, as a general principle, every refugee is an asylum seeker, but not all asylum seekers will successfully become accepted as refugees. Asylum status provides formal recognition as a refugee along with legal protection and material assistance. Many countries have their own procedures for application of asylum status. However, during mass movements of people fleeing conflict or violence, it may not always be possible or necessary to conduct individual interviews with every person. These groups are referred to as "prima facie" refugees. Some have argued for the concept of "survival migration," recognizing the additional violence created by administrative categories and the increased securitization in the process of asylum seeking (Vasey et al. 2016).

For both refugees and asylum seekers, threats to well-being extend across different stages of the migration process, from transit to camps and detention centers, as well as during the application and resettlement periods. Scholars draw on a variety of critical frameworks to highlight the structural vulnerabilities faced by refugees. The concept of structural invisibility (Malkki 1995) has been applied to refugees to describe their noticeable absence in much of the literature on belonging, nations, and nationalism. They are often depicted as a "problem," rather than the result of violence and political oppression that creates massive displacements of people. Refugees are frequently constructed as dangerous and transgressive, blurring what are perceived to be natural boundaries between nation-states. This perception by policymakers and the general public in the receiving country often continues to impact refugees' experiences for many years after their arrival (Becker et al. 2000). Frequently considered suspect, refugees and asylum seekers must often repeatedly prove their worth or experiences of trauma.

A striking feature of recent humanitarian "crises" in Europe and North America is the large number of children and youth seeking asylum. According to UNICEF (2016), over 50 million children have been uprooted worldwide, over half of whom have been forcibly displaced because of conflict. While some journey with family members, others are unaccompanied and travel on their own. Unaccompanied children are defined by the United Nations Human Rights Council as persons younger than 18 years, who have been "separated from both parents and are not being cared for by an adult who, by law or custom, is responsible to do so." Others prefer the term "separated children" as more inclusive of the varied circumstances in which children and youth find themselves without guardianship; this term also emphasizes the social and psychological effects of family separation.

In addition, there are differentially gendered experiences of violence, displacement, and encampment. Women are extremely vulnerable during violent conflicts as well as throughout all phases of the refugee or asylum-seeking experience, and more likely to experience depression, psychosomatic ailments, loneliness, and apathy (Warner 2007). Systematic rape and/or sexual assault is a major feature of militarized conflicts; once they have fled, people may face further gender-based violence in refugee camps and detention centers.

As with other migrant populations, the health of refugees is not only negatively impacted by displacement and resettlement; after all, they enact their mobility in order to flee violent conditions and seek out safety and better opportunities. Research on resilience suggests that factors that encourage positive health outcomes, such as highly supportive living arrangements (Groark et al. 2011; Hodes & Vostanis 2019) and strong social support networks (Zunzunegui et al. 2004), can ameliorate the negative effects of trauma and stress (Arón & Lorion 2003). Resilience refers not just to the absence of ill health but to resources that allow individuals to thrive and overcome adversity, manifesting at the intersection of the personal, biological, and environmental or systemic levels (Almedom & Glandon 2007). Experiences of coping are often also highly gendered, with women often better able to cope due to their roles and responsibilities, whereas men may struggle with downward mobility and effects of unmet gender expectations if they are in exile (e.g., due to lack of employment) (Gideon 2016).

Protracted Displacement: Camps, Sustained Detention, and Reception Centers

Many refugees, such as Somalis or Syrians, are currently living in protracted displacement in neighboring countries of the Global South. As civil wars and violent conflicts force millions from their homes into neighboring countries, these countries are often unprepared to provide adequate housing and medical care. Thus, in contrast to many other types of migrations, developing countries bear the burden, hosting 85% of the world's refugees, with over 27% of the total being provided asylum in the world's least developed countries (UNHCR 2021). This means that already fragile health systems often become overtaxed, presenting challenging situations for host countries.

Health issues in internal displacement camps are often related to overcrowding and inadequate health infrastructure; the ability to offer robust services within these camps is difficult. Many camps have extremely poor sanitary conditions and high population density (Ahoua et al. 2006). One study in the Democratic Republic of the Congo reported the main causes of death to be malnutrition, malaria, infections, and diarrheal diseases (Van Herp et al. 2003). Most illnesses go untreated, especially for reasons of cost (Lori & Boyle 2015). Refugee camps also frequently lack an infrastructure to support vital statistics reporting.

In addition to affecting overall health, social inclusion is greatly impacted by whether refugees are placed in a camp or not. Refugee camps, although they represent spaces of abjectivity, where refugees are excluded from formal political life, also allow people to construct identity, create community, and make claims of citizenship (Redclift 2013a, Redclift 2013b). Camps are both physical and symbolic spaces where personhood is created and reaffirmed, producing and reproducing certain forms of inclusion and exclusion.

Although refugee camps are designed to be places of security, for many they become places of continuing violence, disempowerment, and isolation. The unfavorable conditions in camps may add further stress to the trauma of violence that refugees have experienced in their home countries. For example, a study of displaced Q'eqchi' from Guatemala found that the dispersal of families during the resettlement process separated many women from their natal families, upon whom they depended for social support (Warner 2007). As a result of having no communication with women in their families, there was no one to intervene if they experienced abuse or exploitation by spouses. Furthermore, they experienced disruptions in the transmission of gendered knowledge and skills, thus intensifying the breakdown of social structures.

Beyond camps, which are generally located in third countries, reception centers for refugees in host nations like the one in the opening vignette may also have inadequate conditions, with living spaces lacking sufficient sanitation and safety. This may place people at increased risk for sexual and gender-based violence, especially if they are ill-equipped to manage their own safety due to a lack of information or experience.

In some countries, such as Australia, asylum seekers face mandatory and indefinite detention. Those who arrive by boat are immediately detained in offshore processing centers and are unable to object to or legally challenge this detention. They can be held open-endedly, with 454 days being the average length of time spent in these closed immigration detention centers; about 30% of individuals had been detained more than 2 years (Durham et al. 2016). As a result, Australia is considered to have one of the harshest immigration detention systems in the world, its policy drawing criticism from international organizations as well as health professionals worldwide (Durham et al. 2016). They have charged the Australian government with defying international conventions, denying the human rights of asylum seekers by refusing entry into the country and incarcerating them in a manner that is detrimental to their health (McNeill 2003).

It is now well established that prolonged immigration detention has negative impacts on psychological well-being, including long-term and enduring adverse effects (Hedrick et al. 2020). Health issues treated at Australian detention centers most frequently included dental caries, digestive complaints, respiratory problems, skin lesions, dermatophytosis, ear infections, and upper respiratory tract infections. Prolonged detention was also linked to mental health, musculoskeletal problems, and a variety of dermatological infections, likely the consequence of poor housing conditions (Durham et al. 2016). In addition, numerous deaths by suicide and the rise of self-harm activities appear linked to overcrowding and an increase in length of detention time. This includes higher numbers of people housed inappropriately together, leading to incidents of sexual assault, physical assault, and sexual harassment (Durham et al. 2016).

Medical Examinations and "Proof" of Torture and Persecution

To gain access to refugee status, many applicants must "prove" their claims of torture or persecution as "truth from the body" (Fassin & D'Halluin 2005). Medical certificates – drawn up by a doctor or psychologist to attest to an experience of torture or other trauma – are frequently utilized to this end and are often an essential piece of the asylum application. This turns the body into "a political resource through an expert's mediation" as the body of the refugee becomes a site of inscription of power, as well as of truth, bearing witness to suffering for the institutions of the host country (Fassin & D'Halluin 2005: 598).

Trauma history checklists are frequently employed as a way to standardize refugee mental health experiences and to control for background variables. These measure "frequency," "amount," or "prevalence" of trauma, sometimes reported numerically as a mean with standard deviation, but rarely are able to capture the quality or variety of traumatic events or levels of fear and horror experienced. This focus on measurement means that other relevant factors may be lost, such as context in the home country or during migration (Sigvardsdotter et al. 2016). Furthermore, these checklists have been largely developed in clinical or semiclinical settings, so that there remains a need for more reliable, valid, and culturally acceptable tools for measuring trauma as well as conducting population-level studies (Sigvardsdotter et al. 2016). Asylum seekers are frequently denied refugee status due to caseworkers' lack of knowledge about health issues.

Health Care Access for Refugees and Asylum Seekers

Once refugees and asylum seekers arrive to a permanent host country (or their first country of registration for asylum), access to necessary health care is, in theory, more readily available. In practice, access is often delayed or initially denied. Governments distinguish between these two groups in that asylum seekers have claims for refuge under consideration, while refugees have claims that have been accepted (Thomas 2016). But rights to asylum vary across countries, as do the application processes and their impacts on health care access and quality.

Adapting to life in a host country is made more difficult by fractured and uneven resettlement and integration. For example, in the U.S., resettlement and integration services are supposed to last for five years, but intensive services are only available for three months. After this time, resettlement organizations are no longer required to follow-up with refugees or assist them with job placement or navigating social and health service systems. This is in part because their primary charge is to train them to become economically self-sufficient. However, this idealized American value of self-sufficiency frequently contradicts the fact that refugees are selected for resettlement precisely because of their vulnerability, rather than their ability to achieve financial independence through work (Kerwin 2012). Nonetheless, they are expected to rapidly adapt to life in the U.S., negotiating unfamiliar cultural and social dynamics, while navigating complex material (housing, food, schooling, and transportation) systems. As a result, the U.S. falls well behind other resettlement countries in guaranteeing health equity, in large part due to these competing stressors (Banke-Thomas et al. 2018). The goal of economic self-sufficiency in refugee resettlement policy ultimately places the onus of accessing and affording health care on the individual. In addition, there is an overall lack of appropriate services, which contributes to disparities and poor health outcomes (Clarke et al. 2021).

Many refugees face considerable financial stress because they are obliged to repay the travel expenses incurred during their journeys. To facilitate their travel, they are offered loans by the IOM and required to repay the balance in full within 46 months of resettlement. This obligation – debt accrued on arrival – further impedes the goal of self-sufficiency. Furthermore, the geospatial context may impact their success, as refugees are typically resettled in low-income areas that are commonly underserved by health care institutions and promotion efforts in the first place (Wong et al. 2019).

Where asylum seekers find access to health care may be related to the strength of their social networks (e.g., friends or family members already living in the country), perceived opportunities, or government dispersal processes. For example, Germany and the United Kingdom utilize forced dispersal practices to move asylum seekers to designated spaces. This has been considered problematic because it restricts movement within the host country, disrupts social ties, and affects possibilities for settlement and integration. The use of accommodation or reception centers, as described in the opening vignette, also impacts access to and the effectiveness of health services and can lead to a deterioration of health over time.

Once settled into the temporary or permanent host country, refugees face other significant barriers to service access. These are similar to those described in earlier chapters: language barriers, transportation hurdles, and discrimination. Other disparities may be linked to the policy environment and how access to care is regulated. For example, in Germany, a decentralized governance system and poor clarification of so-called essential services has impeded equitable health care for asylum seekers

(Gottlieb & Schülle 2021). The regulation of restricted health benefits for asylum seekers occurs through a parallel system, separate from statutory health insurance; here, an easy solution to reduce the burden on them would be the integration into Germany's statutory system.

Unique Health Needs of Refugees

Studies on health outcomes for resettled refugees indicate increased rates of communicable and non-communicable diseases, malnutrition, and mental health disorders. There are significant health-related differences by reason for immigration. People who migrate to seek asylum report worse health outcomes compared to those migrating for employment, family, or study reasons (Giuntella et al. 2018). In addition, while there is convergence over time with the health outcomes of native populations for those who migrated for employment, family, or study reasons, the opposite is true for those who seek asylum, for whom ill health persists over time (Giuntella et al. 2018).

There are also vastly different notions of deservingness between refugees and other types of migrants. One U.S.-based study explored the differences in treatment and access to resources between Cuban refugees and other immigrants, revealing divergent conceptions regarding the moral worthiness of each group (Horton 2004). For example, one hospital implemented a pay-up-front policy for undocumented (primarily Mexican) immigrants, while (primarily Cuban) refugees receive welfare and medical benefits for up to eight months, food assistance, job training, and rental aid. In the wake of neoliberal policy reforms, this creates new classes of "deserving" or "undeserving" groups, with the deployment of cultural difference and moral worthiness resulting in persistent inequalities in clinical situations. Horton argues that it becomes the role of civic institutions, including the public health care system, to inculcate normative behavior on behalf of the state; otherwise, some migrant groups may be written off as lost causes, unworthy of attention based often on notions of racialized dispositions. These attributes are commonly associated with "whiteness," such as self-discipline and self-reliance, and used as "popular estimates of a group's economic worth [...and] serve to either 'whiten' or 'blacken' immigrant groups" (Horton 2004: 474). As with other migrant populations discussed in prior chapters, refugees are frequently blamed for bringing disease to the host country. Such misinformation in the press and on social media exaggerating disease risks must be firmly countered with epidemiological data to better inform policymakers and the general public (Khan et al. 2016).

Discordant health beliefs may present an additional challenge for refugees in host countries and may impact patient expectations regarding clinical interactions and treatment. Among Somali refugees in Minnesota, for instance, researchers described the ways in which their health beliefs contrasted sharply with those of clinicians, who relied on the biomedical model that drives medicine in most receiving countries. Their perceptions of health and illness were situated in broader life experiences rather than conceptualized as individually experienced events;

however, the U.S. health care system is fragmented, prioritizing physical over social and mental well-being. Even when women described their explanatory models to health care providers, the health care systems in which they are embedded expect efficiency and do not structure in adequate time to listen or adapt to them (Pavlish et al. 2010). This created frustrations both on the part of patients and their providers and often diminished the perceived quality of health care (Pavlish et al. 2010).

Many refugees combine biomedical and traditional beliefs and healing modalities into pluralistic systems. For example, Cambodian refugees in the U.S. pursue multilevel healing systems, engaging both with medical clinics and indigenous healers (Pickwell 1999). In addition to dealing with loss, psychological distress, and resettlement issues, refugees frequently look for quick and easy access to treat both physical illness and emotional distress. In the case of Cambodian refugees, indigenous healers among them were able to offer familiar remedies, in addition to the services offered by the American medical system (and especially by physicians from Southeast Asia, who were known for their established practices in the community). These "accommodative practitioners," Western-trained Vietnamese physicians, blended different health models into care that was appealing to these refugees, in addition to locating their practices in ethnic neighborhoods to improve accessibility (Pickwell 1999).

Finally, many refugees report shocking levels of food insecurity. In one study among sub-Saharan African refugees, as many as 85% of households lacked food security, because of limited income, difficultly with the English language, and dietary integration issues (McElrone et al. 2019). The last point refers to a variety of issues, including problems accessing, affording, cooking, and shopping for food.

Refugee Mental Health

Displaced populations are at elevated risk of mental health problems, predominantly PTSD. However, the provision of mental health services to refugees and asylum seekers is an overwhelming challenge. In addition, research on this issue is limited and focuses mainly on those in developed countries, which account for less than 20% of displaced persons (Lori & Boyle 2015; Mels et al. 2010).

When displaced, refugees bring their experiences of violence and terror with them, which often becomes embodied as distress. There are two contending approaches regarding the mental health of refugees (Gideon 2016). One uses Western models of trauma and the psychological sequelae of trauma, such as PTSD and depression. However, this approach has been critiqued on two levels. First, it medicalizes distress, so that violence and other events are transformed into micro, medicalized experiences removed from their larger social and political context. Second, this approach fails to acknowledge the other social, political, and economic factors in refugees' lives, focusing on their exposure to violence in the home country to the detriment of other stressors that appear post-migration. This approach leaves little room for defining their own needs and priorities.

Another model suggests that not all distressing experiences become PTSD; it fundamentally questions the Western trauma framework's adequacy by suggesting there are "ordinary" responses to trauma that must be separated from the "extraordinary" ones that require some kind of treatment. It critiques approaches that present refugees as a homogeneous group of passive victims. Instead, there is need for more discussion of the impact of sociodemographic factors (e.g., gender, race, sexuality, class). This perspective also embraces a focus on resilience of refugees, shifting the frame to a salutogenic one and seeking to de-medicalize the issue. Resilience is a dynamic process that has components of "everydayness" to overcome some stressors. Being labeled a "victim" can be stigmatizing and detrimental when, for example, seeking employment as someone labeled as traumatized.

Among refugee children, reports of PTSD prevalence vary widely, with between 20% and 84% demonstrating clinically significant symptoms (Curtis et al. 2018). There is consensus that symptoms increase with the number of traumatic events experienced before and during migration. Children separated from their families are at greater risk of PTSD than accompanied children and face higher levels of depression and anxiety than their peers in the general population. Rates of emotional and mental health distress among refugee children also vary by gender in complex ways and with contradictory findings in the literature – ranging from no differences to higher prevalence of stress, anxiety, and depression among girls (Curtis et al. 2018). One of the conclusions to be drawn is that psychosocial difficulties appear to manifest differently by gender, as well as look different at various ages or life stages. In the literature, girls are described as having more emotional problems and reporting feelings of loneliness, while boys indicate more behavioral problems, with older boys expressing feeling lonely more than younger ones (Curtis et al. 2018).

Social and structural factors in the receiving country have been shown to play a significant role across studies on mental health, with challenges for those experiencing social exclusion or discrimination, those who have limited if any control over their daily lives, or those who struggle to uphold a coherent sense of identity and life purpose. As host country environments have become less welcoming of refugees, experiences of perceived discrimination have increased and further challenged psychological adaptation (Curtis et al. 2018). Uncertain legal status is associated with social and material insecurity; these cumulative stressors, alongside discrimination, worsen mental health over time (Becker et al. 2000; Curtis et al. 2018).

Conclusion

This chapter has explored the unique circumstances of populations that have experienced forced displacement – refugees and asylum seekers – and how these impact health and well-being. Claims of legitimacy and deservingness frequently come into play, and even once (re-)settled, refugees face barriers similar to those described in earlier chapters, including limits to guaranteed access, language issues, and discrimination. Effective solutions need to be more attentive to the larger social, political, economic factors that impact refugees' lives.

The following chapter (Conclusion) summarizes major insights from a critical perspective provided throughout this book and explicates future research needs and strategies to tackle the health inequities that affect migrants.

11
CONCLUSION

As migration continues to be a defining global issue and its impact on health increasingly an area of interest, multiple actors – scholars, medical professionals, NGOs, and governments – are engaged with studying and addressing the issue. This book has called for a radical rethinking of migration and health by critically assessing conventional wisdom and discourse about mobility and bordering processes, as well as how health care systems are inherently unequal systems that function better for some populations than for others. In the following pages, the critical perspective is revisited and implications for improving migrant health are explored. This chapter outlines the search for solutions and suggests future research and policy imperatives.

Moving Forward with a Critical Agenda

This book has laid out some fundamental principles to consider in recognizing or crafting a critical approach to migration and health. These include locating the causes of ill health not in behavioral or cultural factors but rather in structural conditions of inequality – and the larger historical and political processes that underlie those. Migrants experience unique impacts on health due to restricted access to care, systemic constraints related to inequality, poverty, and living and working conditions, as well as the stress associated with precarious legal status. This focus integrates and emphasizes non-medical factors that influence health and considers the broader environments in which immigrants live. Migrants are also frequently excluded precisely because they are located outside the formal system of rights accorded by citizenship and other notions of belonging; this is a specific axis of inequality that remains understudied. However, while some migrants share similar experiences due to their mobility patterns or "illegality," local context impacts the everyday experience of how this shared condition is negotiated.

DOI: 10.4324/9781003307532-11

A critical approach requires explicit attention to the exercise and distribution of social, political, and economic power, along with an acknowledgment that migration is the result of broader colonial and globalization processes that continue to displace populations. The broader historical context of migration must thus be explicitly considered in scholarship on migrant health, including attention to the circumstances that produce the motives for migration, including economic deprivation, social inequality, climate change, political instability, and violence. However, as a global phenomenon and key driver of some forms of development and opportunity, migration can also be a positive experience; though it emerges from inequality, it allows individuals and groups to exercise their agency and fundamental right to access a wider range of resources and may contribute to their well-being.

In investigating migrant health, this book has argued for the inclusion of multiple, diverse, and intersectional standpoints, as well as shifting spatial and temporal influences. A critical approach rejects orderly binary oppositions in favor of alternative vocabularies that acknowledge complex, tangled, temporary, and intermediate experiences, situations, and spaces. This is because migration is not linear, unidirectional, or easily split into discrete "phases," as this implies stabile epistemic partitions between "here" and "there." In addition, migrant experiences must also be conceptualized as intersectional, since health-related opportunities as well as injustices are enacted on a multidimensional basis dependent on factors such as gender, age, country of origin, sexual orientation, skill and education level, and social class.

A critical approach also encourages us to problematize our own standpoint as citizens not only to account for our own positionality and its role in producing intrinsic inequality but also in shaping the analytic lens on the issue of migrant health. As this book has argued, we must be acutely attentive to issues of terminology, because they entail situating oneself in debates on migration and, often, troubling notions of "deservingness." It recommends avoiding the use of violent and militarized terms such as "crisis," or "floods," as well as dehumanizing language such as "illegal immigrant" or "unaccompanied alien minor."

The book reminds us to trouble notions of "borders" and "migration" at every juncture. Rather than referencing borders as naturalized, background objects that are a taken-for-granted (often physical) feature of nation-states, we must recognize them as contingent, shifting, and often violent constructions. They selectively open and close to different groups for reasons that are not logical, fair, or ethical. It also rejects colonialist and ethnocentric thinking that assumes the Global North to always be the preferred destination(s).

A critical approach recognizes human freedom of movement not only as normal and patterned adaption but as a fundamental right, instead of rendering migration as transgressive, exceptional, or pathological. Taking the human rights of migrants seriously also requires us to unsettle commonly circulating ideas and rethink ideas regarding the right to mobility (Estévez 2012). A decolonized global justice underscores the obligations of receiving countries – primarily Western democracies – to respect the rights of migrants, which is ultimately in their own interest.

The exclusion of migrants in host societies is, in fact, not inevitable, although it is the predictable outcome of the securitization of borders (including their internalization and externalization), the criminalization of migrants, the hardening of asylum policy, and the use of increasingly problematic detention and deportation practices.

In our globalized world, no health issue is truly domestic. Migration exemplifies the ways in which disruptions in some parts of the world affect health in others, requiring responses at a global scale. A critical approach recognizes that the health of migrants is significantly impacted by inequality, poverty, institutional constraints, and violence in host countries, rather than an expression of conditions in the countries of origin. In addition, migrant vulnerability shapes the lives of non-migrants and communities connected to them. Thus, policies related to migrants' well-being should be "founded upon a shared humanity, respect for human rights and on the idea that effective public health cannot and should not be confined within the borders and to the citizens of any host country" (Wild & Dawson 2018: 66).

A critical perspective can also suggest fruitful areas of intervention and explicate future research needs and strategies to tackle the health inequities that affect migrants. The remainder of this chapter will explore these possibilities.

The Search for Solutions

The hallmark 1978 Declaration of Alma-Ata, accepted by member countries of the World Health Organization (WHO), expressed the need for action by governments to protect and promote the health of all people. Such action has been woefully inadequate for immigrants around the globe, among other populations. While several international treaties govern issues of migrant health, this global policy arena remains largely uncoordinated and inconsistent. While many (most) nations have signed onto conventions ensuring the right of migrants to health at the level of citizens, these are rarely legally binding and cannot be enforced realistically. For the most part, policies are focused on the isolated national level and do not or are unable to address cross-border issues, lacking the ability for multinational coordination.

As this book has illustrated, immigration involves challenging adaptations to new contexts, but this process occurs at a level beyond the individual and represents a complex and often lengthy negotiation with social, systemic, political, and economic forces. It impacts all other social relationships and has direct effects on health and well-being, not all of which are negative. One implication is that scholars, practitioners, and heath care systems at large must refrain from exceptionalizing migration experiences and instead respond to and integrate them as a usual part of delivery of care. This means, specifically, improvements in physician training and clinical awareness of structural factors leading to illness, adequate availability of interpreters, and a willingness to acknowledge and eliminate other barriers to care. It also means ensuring access to the regular health care system – not a parallel system run by charity efforts – and guaranteeing the ability to file claims for occupational injuries without fear of retribution. Health systems need support in becoming "migration aware" (Wickramage 2018), or what the IOM terms "mobility competent," to recognize human moblity as a central concern for care, research, and policy.

A critical approach thus compels researchers and practitioners to support specific policy and programmatic interventions. These interventions, as this book has stressed, must be at the systemic rather than the individual level. It is easier to pathologize individual behaviors and choices, telling people to eat healthy, exercise, and engage in mental health self-care than it is to focus on systemic, structural issues that fundamentally constrain these kinds of activities. However, there remains a lack of coordinated efforts to address the known health inequities that migrants experience globally, in addition to glaring inconsistencies between migration patterns and the responses of policymakers. For instance, this book has highlighted the fact that, although epidemiological studies indicate that migrants are often among the most disadvantaged when it comes to health, empirical evidence also shows that even in nations with universal health care systems, migrants generally have lower rates of utilization, and unauthorized migrants have little to no access to care at all. Therefore, it makes little sense to formally exclude them. Furthermore, their access opportunities must be based on entitlement, rather than notions of charity, deservingness, or luck. Many of the examples presented in the book in which migrants were able to access care make reference to how people described this good fortune: Dr. Ramirez in Chapter 3 described migrants who found their way to his small office in the migrant shelter in Mazatlán, Mexico as "lucky," because they had survived their treacherous journeys thus far; Javier in Chapter 5 described how his siblings were "lucky" to be born in the U.S. as the only ones with adequate access to the health care system; and Sarah in Chapter 8, the Ghanaian women living in Berlin, framed as "lucky" her opportunity to get a bed in the hospital where she would deliver her baby. Complacency and reliance on luck is the opposite of ensuring access to health services based on fundamental human rights.

Finally, as some have argued, a critical approach must "take as its first premise the priority and prerogative of the elemental and elementary human freedom of movement" (De Genova 2016: 236). As a result of the violences caused by borders, some scholars and physicians have advocated for their abolition altogether as an important site of medical intervention. Rather than tacitly accept the modern system of borders, refusal is an important step in genuine solidarity with migrants by "challenging global infrastructures that drive displacement" (Dubal et al. 2021: 1).

Future Research Imperatives

It is a crucial time to speculate the research and advocacy priorities for migrant health, which also will require a more enabling environment than is currently in existence at national, regional, and global levels in order to develop evidence-based inter-sectoral policies and priority setting processes (Wickramage et al. 2018).

Immigration status, as we have seen, can impact health through several mechanisms, including differential access to resources, stress, and poor labor and housing conditions. There remains a lack of focus on the explicit role of discrimination as it plays out through racialization processes, racism, prejudice, and anti-immigrant violence. These factors are known to impact both mental and physical health and are likely more important in the health outcomes of migrants than previously recognized, necessitating additional research and policy attention.

Other specific topical areas remain understudied, such as undocumented migrants' access to expensive but lifesaving care (e.g., major surgeries or transplants), clinical ethics and practical decision-making by health care workers and administrators, reproductive politics, dental/oral health, and public health threats generated by the denial of health care to unauthorized im/migrants. As border control and law enforcement activities continue to increase in host countries, researchers must examine how migrants' "policeability" impacts health outcomes. Processes of illegality produce conditions that maintain the vulnerability of im/migrants, creating a disjuncture between physical and legal presence and creating a "space of nonexistence" (Coutin 2003). The violent effects of border regimes remain to be adequately addressed.

In addition to larger national policies that exclude or criminalize migrants, we must be attentive to scale and investigate the impacts of specific local policies. For example, many cities, provinces, and states have adopted explicit rights for farmworker organizing, put into place minimum wages for workers in the service industry, offered opportunities for irregular migrants to obtain identification cards or driver's licenses, and implemented policies for educational access for migrant children. Studies should account for such localized circumstances, striving for deeper understanding of a specific policy's impact rather than seeking to make broad generalizations for all immigrant populations.

One major imperative is that research *about* migrants needs to be conducted *by* and/or *with* migrants. Traditional research methods rarely attempt to employ marginalized peoples' knowledge. Instead, new approaches and commitments are needed. This can include community-based and participatory approaches with migrant communities, but also compels their training and inclusion in, for example, the academy, as researchers and practitioners. Bi- or multinational approaches to understanding migrant health can offer additional critical insights, including a wider range of health-related topics, an increase in research that examines connections between transnational or binational communities, greater exploration of chronic disease risk factors, and more detailed investigations into the migration experience itself.

There are several areas where more voices need to be heard. There is a lack of research, for example, that privileges the expressions of migrant children themselves to better understand their complex health needs (Curtis et al. 2018). At the other end of the temporal spectrum, few researchers have examined end of life among migrants and what happens in their social worlds; we need more understandings of mobility among the elderly; return to home countries upon retirement and with disability; migration-sensitive palliative care; and processes of final bodily repatriation.

In addition, immigration impacts the health of non-immigrants. For example, this book noted that in the U.S., most children living in 2.3 million mixed-status families are U.S. citizens by birth. They are directly affected by the undocumented status of their family members; they access health care benefits at a lower rate or receive delayed treatment, experience greater developmental risk in childhood, and experience higher levels of family conflict and stress, including the effects of deportation of individual household members, often parents. In addition, children are often left behind in the community of origin and experience negative effects of familial separation. These situations underscore the fact that migrants are embedded in social units, creating a cumulative ripple effect on households and wider communities. This has important implications for the health impacts of policies that restrict family reunification for growing immigrant and refugee populations around the globe. Related to this, immigrant legal status must be understood as a fluid characteristic that can change – often multiple times – over the course of an individual's lifetime owing to personal circumstances (e.g., marriage) and shifting policy environments (e.g., legalization).

There should also be a greater focus on resiliency. Resiliency, or the ability of a population to respond positively despite factors challenging its health, represents a strengths-based approach as opposed to the more common deficit focus in research. However, resiliency is used frequently in the well-being literature as something that an individual has or can develop to make them more able to cope; this concept can be critiqued for taking the focus off structural issues and placing it onto individuals. Thus, it is important to focus on the resiliency of a *population* or a *community,* rather than at the individual level. This requires rethinking risk and vulnerability in the context of marginalized populations, and specifically requires the disruption of disabling structures and processes, as well as the re-imagining of communities, relationships, social spaces, and representations in the context of scarce power resources (Hutcheon & Lashewicz 2014). This is particularly salient for migrant populations, who are highly marginalized at the same time as their experiences are often lumped together despite diverse experiences, histories, and statuses. A critical approach to resiliency thus interrogates pathogenic structures and processes that impact well-being to unsettle and ultimately replace them, in addition to focusing analyses on social capital, informal care networks, and community resistance to policies and practices detrimental to health. Taking seriously the resiliency of migrants suggests a commitment to working with communities not only to understand their needs but also to identify and build on their strengths.

As noted in the introduction to this book, in addition to the mobility of populations, *immobility* has become an important feature of contemporary migration. We still need a better understanding about the health impacts of immobility for people who do not have the resources, assets, or networks to migrate, as well as for those who choose to remain behind for reasons of place attachment or sociocultural continuity. Many of these immobile populations are living in sites of extreme climate vulnerability and may increasingly experience adverse health impacts related to water and food insecurity, changes in disease ecology, flooding and saltwater intrusion, and the psychosocial impacts of disrupted livelihoods (McMichael 2020).

Indeed, in the future, climate change will increasingly impact patterns of migration, amplifying contributory and proximate causes of displacement and increasing pressures on various communities and regions. These include both slow-onset changes (e.g., food insecurity related to drought, sea-level rise) and fast-onset changes such as extreme weather (McMichael 2020). Increased migration will continue to be a strategic and adaptive response to these anthropogenic environmental shifts; some have even argued for a radical change in perspective so that human mobility is seen as part of the solution rather than part of the problem (Tacoli 2009). This will require policymakers to carefully consider the role of local and national institutions in supporting and accommodating mobility. At the same time, it does not address the underlying inequalities that lead the world's wealthier populations to produce vast quantities of greenhouse gasses that make the less wealthy suffer the greatest impacts of climate change, requiring them to be on the move.

What will a research agenda for the study of migration and health look like post-pandemic? Will global migration flows slow down or speed up? How and why? Migration scholars are accustomed to studying people on the move along with the state responses to this movement. However, the pandemic's effect on migrant communities has been characterized more by immobility than by movement, requiring a shift in focus. Although some migrants returned to their home countries, many others were stranded by travel restrictions and border closures, either in destination countries, zones of transit, or by having been unable to move abroad as intended. Thus, a theoretical and practical focus on the effects of forced immobility has become high priority. In addition, a global drop in remittances had severe effects for families, communities, and countries worldwide. As this threatens the well-being of communities and countries of origin, it also calls into question the linkages between migration and development that underlie much of international cooperation on the issue.

Furthermore, discourses about protecting public health seem poised to replace securitization narratives that emerged post-9/11 for governments seeking to strengthen their external borders and limit immigration. Will public health increasingly be used as a rationale not only to control border crossings but to further disenfranchise communities post-migration? Over the past decades, we have seen a respatialization of borders, which, through technologies of surveillance, now often appear to be both everywhere and nowhere at the same time. How will responses to pandemics further push borders into the interior and allow them to transcend physical boundaries? What will be the impacts on immigrant communities, especially as they interplay with intensified surveillance and exclusionary policies?

One of the lasting impacts of the pandemic will be that it has prompted new migration as people's livelihoods are affected and their communities flattened by the social, demographic, and economic impacts. With increasing and widespread displacement around the globe, the search for long-lasting solutions for refugees and asylum seekers will become more acute than ever. As governments prioritize pressing public health, economic, and other domestic considerations, will the Global Compact for Safe, Orderly, and Regular Migration and other treaties be able to meet the test of a changed era? These are some of the important considerations moving forward as we take stock of the field of migration and health, especially as pandemics have once again underscored the central importance of human mobility, interconnections across borders, and the persistence of social and economic inequality around the globe.

Migrants, it has been said, are the "canaries in the coal mine" (Lee et al. 2018) of social equality, and a society's treatment of this group, especially when it comes to health, is a barometer for how well it treats all other marginalized populations. A critical approach is, ultimately, one that is committed to eliminating health disparities and uplifting migrant populations.

REFERENCES

Abraído-Lanza, A. F., Chao, M. T., & Flórez, K. R. (2005). Do healthy behaviors decline with greater acculturation? Implications for the Latino mortality paradox. *Social Science & Medicine*, 61, 1243–1255.

Abrego, L. J. (2014). *Sacrificing families: Navigating laws, labor, and love across borders*. Stanford University Press.

Abrego, L. J., & Lakhani, S. M. (2015). Incomplete inclusion: Legal violence and immigrants in liminal legal statuses. *Law & Policy*, 37(4), 265–293.

Abrego, L. J., & Menjívar, C. (2011). Immigrant Latina mothers as targets of legal violence. *International Journal of Sociology of the Family*, 37(1), 9–26.

Acevedo-Garcia, D., & Bates, L. M. (2007). Latino health paradoxes: Empirical evidence, explanations, future research, and implications. In H. Rodríguez, R. Sáenz, & C. Menjívar (Eds.), *Latinas/os in the United States: Changing the face of America* (pp. 101–113). Springer.

Adams, A., Realpe, A., Vail, L., Buckingham, C. D., Erby, L. H., & Roter, D. (2015). How doctors' communication style and race concordance influence African-Caribbean patients when disclosing depression. *Patient Education & Counseling*, 98(10), 1266–1273.

Afulani, P. A., Torres, J. M., Sudhinaraset, M., & Asunka, J. (2016). Transnational ties and the health of sub-Saharan African migrants: The moderating role of gender and family separation. *Social Science & Medicine*, 168, 63–71.

Agadjanian, V., Arnaldo, C., & Cau, B. (2011). Health costs of wealth gains: Labor migration and perceptions of HIV/AIDS risks in Mozambique. *Social Forces*, 89 (4), 1097–1117.

Agudelo-Suárez, A., Gil-Gonzalez, D., Ronda-Pérez, E., Porthe, V., Paramio-Perez, G., García, A. M., & Garí, A. (2009). Discrimination, work and health in immigrant populations in Spain. *Social Science & Medicine*, 68(10), 1866–1874.

Ahoua, L., Tamrat, A., Duroch, F., Grais, R. F., & Brown, V. (2006). High mortality in an internally displaced population in Ituri, Democratic Republic of Congo, 2005: Results of a rapid assessment under difficult conditions. *Global Public Health*, 1(3), 195–204.

Alcántara, C., Chen, C. N., & Alegría, M. (2015a). Transnational ties and past-year major depressive episodes among Latino immigrants. *Cultural Diversity and Ethnic Minority Psychology*, 21(3), 486.

Alcántara, C., Molina, K. M., & Kawachi, I. (2015b). Transnational, social, and neighborhood ties and smoking among Latino immigrants: Does gender matter? *American Journal of Public Health*, 105(4), 741–749.

Alexander, W. L., & Fernandez, M. (2014). Immigration policing and medical care for farmworkers: Uncertainties and anxieties in the East Coast migrant stream. *North American Dialogue*, 17(1), 13–30.

Alioua, M. (2017). Transnational migration is always a migration in stages: The Moroccan stopover of sub-Saharan migration. In L.-A. Bernes, H. Bousetta, & C. Zickgraf (Eds.), *Migration in the Western Mediterranean* (pp. 139–160). Routledge.

Allen, B., Cisneros, E. M., & Tellez, A. (2015). The children left behind: The impact of parental deportation on mental health. *Journal of Child and Family Studies*, 24(2), 386–392.

Almedom, A. M., & Glandon, D. (2007). Resilience is not the absence of PTSD any more than health is the absence of disease. *Journal of Loss and Trauma*, 12(2), 127–143.

Alpes, G. (2020). *Emergency returns by IOM from Libya and Niger: A protection response or a source of protection concerns?* Medico International.

Altenburg, F. (2012). Health services for undocumented migrants in Europe: An overview. In G. Biffl & F. Altenburg (Eds.), *Migration and health in Nowhereland: Access of undocumented migrants to work and health care in Europe* (pp. 99–108). Omninum.

Alunni, L. (2015). Securitarian healing: Roma mobility and health care in Rome. *Medical Anthropology*, 34(2), 139–149.

Amon, J. J., & Todrys, K. W. (2008). Fear of foreigners: HIV-related restrictions on entry, stay, and residence. *Journal of the International AIDS Society*, 11(1), 1–6.

Anarfi, J. K., Kwnaky, S. O., & Ahiadeke, C. (2005). Migration, return and impact in Ghana. In T. Manuh (Ed.), *At home in the world: International migration and development in contemporary Ghana and West Africa* (pp. 204–226). Sub-Saharan Publishers.

Andersson, R. (2014a). *Illegality, Inc.: Clandestine migration and the business of bordering Europe*. University of California Press.

Andersson, R. (2014b). Time and the migrant other: European border controls and the temporal economics of illegality. *American Anthropologist*, 116(4), 795–809.

Androff, D. K., Ayon, C., Becerra, D., & Gurrola, M. (2011). U.S. immigration policy and immigrant children's well-being: The impact of policy shifts. *Journal of Sociology & Social Welfare*, 38, 77.

Antecol, H., & Bedard, K. (2006). Unhealthy assimilation: Why do immigrants converge to American health status levels? *Demography*, 43, 337–360.

Arbona, C., Olvera, N., Rodriguez, N., Hagan, J., Linares, A., & Wiesner, M. (2010). Acculturative stress among documented and undocumented Latino immigrants in the United States. *Hispanic Journal of Behavioral Sciences*, 32(3), 362–384.

Arcury, T. A., Grzywacz, J. G., Sidebottom, J., & Wiggins, M. F. (2013). Overview of immigrant worker occupational health and safety for the agriculture, forestry, and fishing (AgFF) sector in the southeastern United States. *American Journal of Industrial Medicine*, 56(8), 911–924.

Arcury, T. A., O'Hara, H., Grzywacz, J. G., Isom, S., Chen, H., & Quandt, S. A. (2012). Work safety climate, musculoskeletal discomfort, working while injured, and depression among migrant farmworkers in North Carolina. *American Journal of Public Health*, 102(S2), S272–S278.

Armenta, A. (2017). Racializing crimmigration: Structural racism, colorblindness, and the institutional production of immigrant criminality. *Sociology of Race and Ethnicity*, 3(1), 82–95.

Arón, A. M., & Lorion, R. P. (2003). A case report of a community-based response to domestic violence in Chile. *Journal of Community Psychology*, 31(6), 561–579.

Asch, S., Frayne, S., & Waitzkin, H. (1995). To discharge or not to discharge: Ethics of care for an undocumented immigrant. *Journal of Health Care for the Poor and Underserved*, 6(1), 3–9.

Asch, S., Leake, B., Anderson, R., & Gelberg, L. (1998). Why do symptomatic patients delay obtaining care for tuberculosis? *American Journal of Respiratory and Critical Care Medicine*, 157(4), 1244–1248.

Babahaji, L. (2020). *The current state of migrant health in Morocco: Pre-and peri-COVID-19 pandemic*. Independent Study Project (ISP) Collection. 3353. https://digitalcollections.sit.edu/isp_collection/3353

Bachelet, S. (2019). "Looking for one's life": Trapped mobilites and adventure in Morocco. *Migration and Society*, 2(1), 40–54.

Baird, T., & van Liempt, I. (2016). Scrutinising the double disadvantage: Knowledge production in the messy field of migrant smuggling. *Journal of Ethnic and Migration Studies*, 42(3), 400–417.

Balaguera, M. (2018). Trans-migrations: Agency and confinement at the limits of sovereignty. Signs: *Journal of Women in Culture and Society*, 43(3), 641–664.

Balaguera, M. (2019). *Citizenship in transit: Perils and promises of crossing Mexico*. PhD dissertation, University of Massachusetts, Amherst.

Balcazar, H., Castro, F. G., & Krull, J. L. (1995). Cancer risk reduction in Mexican American women: The role of acculturation, education, and health risk factors. *Health Education Quarterly*, 22(1), 61–84.

Banati, P. (2007). Risk amplification: HIV in migrant communities. *Development South Africa*, 24(1), 205–223.

Banke-Thomas, A., Agbemenu, K., & Johnson-Agbakwu, C. (2019). Factors associated with access to maternal and reproductive health care among Somali refugee women resettled in Ohio, United States: A cross-sectional survey. *Journal of Immigrant and Minority Health*, 21(5), 946–953.

Bärnighausen, T., Hosegood, V., Timaeus, I. M., & Newell, M. L. (2007). The socioeconomic determinants of HIV incidence: Evidence from a longitudinal, population-based study in rural South Africa. *AIDS*, 21(7), S29–S38.

Basok, T., Bélanger, D., Rojas Wiesner, M. L., & Candiz, G. (2015). *Rethinking transit migration: Precarity, mobility, and self-making in Mexico*. Palgrave Macmillan.

Baum, J. (2010). *In the child's best interest? The consequences of losing a lawful immigrant parent to deportation*. DIANE Publishing.

Beardwood, B. A., Kirsh, B., & Clark, N. J. (2005). Victims twice over: Perceptions and experiences of injured workers. *Qualitative Health Research*, 15(1), 30–48.

Becerra, D., Androff, D., Cimino, A., Alex Wagaman, M., & Blanchard, K. N. (2013). The impact of perceived discrimination and immigration policies upon perceptions of quality of life among Latinos in the U.S. *Race and Social Problems*, 5(1), 65–78.

Becker, G., Beyene, Y., & Ken, P. (2000). Memory, trauma, and embodied distress: The management of disruption in the stories of Cambodians in exile. *Ethos*, 28(3), 320–345.

Benjet, C., Borges, G., Medina-Mora, M. E., Zambrano, J., & Aguilar-Gaxiola, S. (2009). Youth mental health in a populous city of the developing world: Results from the Mexican Adolescent Mental Health Survey. *Journal of Child Psychology and Psychiatry*, 50(4), 386–395.

Benson, P. (2008). El Campo: Faciality and structural violence in farm labor camps. *Cultural Anthropology*, 23(4), 589–629.

Berk, M. L., & Schur, C. L. (2001). The effect of fear on access to care among undocumented Latino immigrants. *Journal of Immigrant Health*, 3(3), 151–156.

Berk, M. L., Schur, C. L., Chavez, L. R., & Frankel, M. (2000). Health care use among undocumented Latino immigrants: Is free health care the main reason why Latinos come to the United States? A unique look at the facts. *Health Affairs*, 19(4), 51–64.

Berriane, M., De Haas, H., & Natter, K. (2015). Introduction: Revisiting Moroccan migrations. *The Journal of North African Studies*, 20(4), 503–521.

Bialasiewicz, L. (2012). Off-shoring and out-sourcing the borders of Europe: Libya and EU border work in the Mediterranean. *Geopolitics*, 17(4), 843–866.

Bilger, V., Hollomey, C., Efionayi-Mäder, D., & Wyssmüller, C. (2011). *Health care for undocumented migrants in Switzerland: Policies, people, practices*. International Center for Migration Policy Development.

Biswas, D., Kristiansen, M., Krasnik, A., & Norredam, M. (2011). Access to healthcare and alternative health-seeking strategies among undocumented migrants in Denmark. *BMC Public Health*, 11(1), 1–11.

Blanchard, J., Nayar, S., & Lurie, N. (2007). Patient-provider and patient-staff racial concordance and perceptions of mistreatment in the health care setting. *Journal of General Internal Medicine*, 22(8), 1184–1189.

Boden, L. I., Biddle, E. A., & Spieler, E. A. (2001). Social and economic impacts of workplace illness and injury: Current and future directions for research. *American Journal of Industrial Medicine*, 40(4), 398–402.

Boehm, D. A. (2011). Here/not here: Contingent citizenship and transnational Mexican children. In C. Coe, R. R. Reynolds, D. A. Boehm, J. M. Hess, & H. Rae-Espinoza (Eds.), Everyday ruptures: Children, youth, and migration in global perspective (pp. 161–173). Vanderbilt University Press.

Boehm, D. A. (2012). *Intimate migrations: Gender, family, and illegality among transnational Mexicans*. New York University Press.

Boehm, D. (2016). *Returned: Going and coming in an age of deportation*. University of California Press.

Bonilla, Y. (2017). Unsettling sovereignty. *Cultural Anthropology*, 32, 330–339.

Boss, P. (2006). *Loss, trauma, and resilience: Therapeutic work with ambiguous loss*. W. W. Norton.

Bourgois, P., & Schonberg, J. (2009). *Righteous dopefiend*. University of California Press.

Bowen, S. (2001). *Language barriers in access to health care*. Health Canada.

Bowlby, J., & Ainsworth, M. (2013). The origins of attachment theory. *Attachment Theory: Social, Developmental, and Clinical Perspectives*, 45, 759–775.

Brabeck, K., & Xu, Q. (2010). The impact of detention and deportation on Latino immigrant children and families: A quantitative exploration. *Hispanic Journal of Behavioral Sciences*, 32(3), 341–361.

Brabeck, K. M., Lykes, M. B., & Hershberg, R. (2011). Framing immigration to and deportation from the U.S.: Central American immigrants make meaning of their experiences. *Community, Work, & Family*, 13(3), 275–296.

Brabeck, K. M., Lykes, M. B., & Hunter, C. (2014). The psychosocial impact of detention and deportation on U.S. migrant children and families. *American Journal of Orthopsychiatry*, 84(5), 496–505.Braveman, P., Egerter, S., & Williams, D. R. (2011). The social determinants of health: Coming of age. *Annual Review of Public Health*, 32, 381–398.

Brotherton, D. C., & Barrios, L. (2011). *Banished to the homeland: Dominican deportees and their stories of exile*. Columbia University Press.

Brouwer, K. C., Lozada, R., Cornelius, W. A., Cruz, M. F., Magis-Rodriguez, C., De Nuncio, M. Z., & Strathdee, S. A. (2009). Deportation along the U.S.–Mexico border: Its relation to drug use patterns and accessing care. *Journal of Immigrant and Minority Health*, 11(1), 1–6.

Brown, P. J., & Closser, S. (2016). *Understanding and applying medical anthropology*. Routledge.

Bryant-Davis, T., & Tummala-Narra, P. (2017). Cultural oppression and human trafficking: Exploring the role of racism and ethnic bias. *Women & Therapy*, 40(1–2), 152–169.

Byaruhanga, R. (2020). The impact of Covid-19 on securitisation of migration and mobility in the United States. *European Journal of Social Sciences Studies*, 5(6). www.oapub.org/soc/index.php/EJSSS/article/view/939. Date accessed: 09 April 2022. DOI: http://dx.doi.org/10.46827/ejsss.v5i6.939.

Caballero, B. (2007). The global epidemic of obesity: An overview. *Epidemiologic reviews*, 29(1), 1–5.

Cairney, J., & Østbye, T. (1999). Time since immigration and excess body weight. *Canadian Journal of Public Health*, 90(2), 120–124.

Calain-Watanabe, T., & Lee, S. (2012). Access to maternal and child care for undocumented migrants in Japan. *Kokusai Hoken Iryo (Journal of International Health)*, 27(3), 207–212.

Capps, R., Castañeda, R. M., Chaudry, A., & Santos, R. (2007). *Paying the price: The impact of immigration raids on America's children*. The Urban Institute. National Council of La Raza. www.urban.org/UploadedPDF/411566_immigration_raids.pdf

Carballo, M., & Nerukar, A. (2001). Migration, refugees, and health risks. *Emerging Infectious Diseases*, 7(3 Suppl.), 556.

Carling, J. (2007). Migration control and migrant fatalities at the Spanish-African borders. *International Migration Review*, 41(2), 316–343.

Carling, J. (2014). Scripting remittances: Making sense of money transfers in transnational relationships. *International Migration Review*, 48, S218–S262.

Carling, J., Menjívar, C., & Schmalzbauer, L. (2012). Central themes in the study of transnational parenthood. *Journal of Ethnic and Migration Studies*, 38(2), 191–217.

Carpenter-Song, E., Nordquest, M., & Longhofer, J. (2007). Cultural competence reexamined: Critique and directions for the future. *Psychiatric Services*, 58, 1362–1365.

Carpiano, R. M. (2006). Toward a neighborhood resource-based theory of social capital for health: Can Bourdieu and sociology help? *Social Science & Medicine*, 62(1), 165–175.

Carrillo, H. (2004). Sexual migration, cross-cultural sexual encounters, and sexual health. *Sexuality Research & Social Policy*, 1(3), 58–70.

Cartwright, E. (2011). Immigrant dreams: Legal pathologies and structural vulnerabilities along the immigration continuum. *Medical Anthropology*, 30(5), 475–495.

Castañeda, H. (2008). Paternity for sale: Anxieties over "demographic theft" and undocumented migrant reproduction in Germany. *Medical Anthropology Quarterly*, 22(4), 340–359.

Castañeda, H. (2009). Illegality as risk factor: A survey of unauthorized migrant patients in a Berlin clinic. *Social Science & Medicine*, 68(8), 1552–1560.

Castañeda, H. (2011). Medical humanitarianism and physicians' organized efforts to provide aid to unauthorized migrants in Germany. *Human Organization*, 70(1), 1–10.

Castañeda, H. (2012). "Over-foreignization" or "unused potential"? A critical review of migrant health in Germany and responses toward unauthorized migration. *Social Science & Medicine*, 74(6), 830–838.

Castañeda, H. (2013). Medical aid as protest: Acts of citizenship for unauthorized im/migrants and refugees. *Citizenship Studies*, 17(2), 227–240.

Castañeda, H. (2019). *Borders of belonging: Struggles and solidarity in mixed-status immigrant families*. Stanford University Press.

Castañeda, H., Holmes, S. M., Madrigal, D. S., DeTrinidad Young, M.-E., Beyerle, N., & James Quesada, J. (2015). Immigration as a social determinant of health. *Annual Review of Public Health*, 36, 75–392.

Castañeda, H., Kline, N., & Dickey, N. (2010). Health concerns of migrant backstretch workers at horse racetracks. *Journal of Health Care for the Poor and Underserved*, 21(2), 489–503.

Castañeda, H., & Melo, M. A. (2014). Health care access for Latino mixed-status families: Barriers, strategies, and implications for reform. *American Behavioral Scientist*, 58(14), 1891–1909.

Castañeda, H., & Melo, M. A. (2019). Geographies of confinement for immigrant youth: Checkpoints and immobilities along the U.S./Mexico border. *Law & Policy*, 41(1), 80–102.

Castillo, C. G. (2018). What the doctors don't see: Physicians as gatekeepers, injured Latino immigrants, and workers' compensation system. *Anthropology of Work Review*, 39(2), 94–104.

Cavazos-Rehg, P. A., Zayas, L. H., & Spitznagel, E. L. (2007). Legal status, emotional well-being and subjective health status of Latino immigrants. *Journal of the National Medical Association*, 99(10), 1126.

Čebron, U. L. (2010). The construction of a health uninsurant: People without medical citizenship as seen by some Slovene health workers. *Studia ethnologica croatica*, 22, 187–212.

Chacón, J. A., & Davis, M. (2006). *No one is illegal: Fighting racism and state violence on the U.S.-Mexico border* (Kindle ed.). Haymarket Books.

Chamberlain, K., & Lyons, A. (2020). Critical and qualitative approaches to behavior change. In M. S. Hagger, L. D. Cameron, K. Hamilton, N. Hankonen and T. Lintunen (Eds.), *The handbook of behavior change* (pp. 430–442). Cambridge University Press.

Chamberlain, K., & Lyons, A. (Eds.). (2021). *Routledge international handbook of critical issues in health and illness.* Routledge.

Chamberlain, M. (2006). *Family love in the diaspora: Migration and the Anglo-Caribbean experience.* Routledge.

Chaudry, A., Capps, R., Pedroza, J. M., Castaneda, R. M., Santos, R., & Scott, M. M. (2010). *Facing our future: Children in the aftermath of immigration enforcement.* Urban Institute.

Chavez, L. R. (1992). *Shadowed lives: Undocumented immigrants in American society*. Harcourt, Brace, Jovanovich.

Chavez, L. R. (2003). Immigration and medical anthropology. N. Foner (Ed.), American arrivals: Anthropology engages the new immigration (pp. 197–227). SAR Press.

Chavez, L. R. (2004). A glass half empty: Latina reproduction and public discourse. *Human Organization*, 63(2), 173–188.

Chavez, L. R. (2017). *Anchor babies and the challenge of birthright citizenship*. Stanford University Press.

Chishti, M., & Bolter, J. (2020). Vulnerable to COVID-19 and in frontline jobs, immigrants are mostly shut out of U.S. relief. Migration Policy Institute. www.migrationpolicy.org/article/covid19-immigrants-shut-out-federal-relief

Clarke, S. K., Kumar, G. S., Sutton, J., Atem, J., Banerji, A., Brindamour, M., … Zaaeed, N. (2021). Potential impact of COVID-19 on recently resettled refugee populations in the United States and Canada: Perspectives of refugee healthcare providers. *Journal of Immigrant and Minority Health*, 23(1), 184–189.

Coe, C. (2021). *Changes in care: Aging, migration, and social class in West Africa*. Rutgers University Press.

Coe, C., Reynolds, R. R., Boehm, D.A., Hess, J. M., & Rae-Espinoza, H. (Eds.). (2011). *Everyday ruptures: Children, youth, and migration in global perspective.* Vanderbilt University Press.

Coker, R. (2004). Compulsory screening of immigrants for tuberculosis and HIV. *BMJ*, 328(7435), 298–300.

Coleman, M. (2012). The "local" migration state: The site-specific devolution of immigration enforcement in the U.S. South. *Law & Policy*, 34(2), 159–190.

Colen, S. (2009). Stratified reproduction and West Indian childcare workers and employers in New York. In E. Lewin (Ed.), Feminist anthropology: A reader (p. 380). Wiley Blackwell.

Collyer, M. (2007). In-between places: Trans-Saharan transit migrants in Morocco and the fragmented journey to Europe. *Antipode*, 39(4), 668–690.

Collyer, M. (2010). Stranded migrants and the fragmented journey. *Journal of Refugee Studies*, 23(3), 273–293.

Cordero, A. L. H. (2021). Mothers who cross borders: Family care networks in the homes of immigrant mothers. In M. Montero-Sieburth, R. M. Giralt, N. Garcia-Arjona, J. Eguren (Eds.), *Family practices in migration* (pp. 138–153). Routledge.

Coutin, S. B. (2000). *Legalizing moves: Salvadoran immigrants' struggle for U.S. residency*. University of Michigan Press.

Coutin, S. B. (2003). *Legalizing moves: Salvadoran immigrants' struggle for U.S. residency*. University of Michigan Press.

Coutin, S. B. (2010). Confined within: National territories as zones of confinement. *Political Geography*, 29(4), 200–208.

Coutin, S. B., Ashar, S. M., Chacón, J. M., & Lee, S. (2017). Deferred action and the discretionary state: Migration, precarity and resistance. *Citizenship Studies*, 21(8), 951–968.

Cristancho, S., Garces, D. M., Peters, K. E., & Mueller, B. C. (2008). Listening to rural Hispanic immigrants in the Midwest: A community-based participatory assessment of major barriers to health care access and use. *Qualitative Health Research*, 18(5), 633–646.

Cupertino, A. P., Suarez, N., Cox, L. S., Fernández, C., Jaramillo, M. L., Morgan, A., … Ellerbeck, E. F. (2013). Empowering promotores de salud to engage in community-based participatory research. *Journal of Immigrant & Refugee Studies*, 11(1), 24–43.

Curtis, P., Thompson, J., & Fairbrother, H. (2018). Migrant children within Europe: A systematic review of children's perspectives on their health experiences. *Public Health*, 158, 71–85.

Czaika M., & Haas, H. (2014). The globalization of migration: Has the world become more migratory? *International Migration Review*, 48(2), 283–323.

Danz, S. M. (2000). A nonpublic forum or a brutal bureaucracy? Advocates' claims of access to welfare center waiting rooms. *New York University Law Review*, 75(4), 1004–1044.

Davis, R. C., & Henderson, N. J. (2003). Willingness to report crimes: The role of ethnic group membership and community efficacy. *Crime & Delinquency*, 49(4), 564–580.

De Genova, N. (2002). Migrant "illegality" and deportability in everyday life. *Annual Review of Anthropology*, 31, 419–447.

De Genova, N. (2013). The securitarian society of the spectacle. In *Rhetorics of Insecurity* (pp. 213–242). New York University Press.

De Genova, N. (2016). The "native's point of view" in the anthropology of migration. *Anthropological Theory*, 16(2–3), 227–240.

De Genova, N., & Peutz, N. (2010). *The deportation regime: Sovereignty, space, and the freedom of movement*. Duke University Press.

De Haas, H. (2007). *The myth of invasion: Irregular migration from West Africa to the Maghreb and the European Union*. International Migration Institute, University of Oxford.

De León, J. (2015). *The land of open graves: Living and dying on the migrant trail*. University of California Press.

Delva, J., Horner, P., Martinez, R., Sanders, L., Lopez, W. D., & Doering-White, J. (2013). Mental health problems of children of undocumented parents in the United States: A hidden crisis. *Journal of Community Positive Practices*, 3, 25–35.

Dembe, A. E. (2001). The social consequences of occupational injuries and illnesses. *American Journal of Industrial Medicine*, 40(4), 403–417.

Desgrees-du-Lou, A., Pannetier, J., Ravalihasy, A., Le Guen, M., Gosselin, A., Panjo, H., … PARCOURS Study Group. (2016). Is hardship during migration a determinant of HIV infection? Results from the ANRS PARCOURS study of sub-Saharan African migrants in France. *AIDS*, 30(4), 645.

Dickson, A. (2015). Distancing asylum seekers from the state: Australia's evolving political geography of immigration and border control. *Australian Geographer*, 46(4), 437–454.

Digidiki, V., & Bhabha, J. (2017). *Emergency within an emergency: The growing epidemic of sexual exploitation and abuse of migrant children in Greece*. Harvard University FXB Center for Health and Human Rights. https://cdn2. sph. harvard. edu/wp-content/uploads/sites/ 5/2017/04/Emergency-Within-an-Emergency-FXB. pdf

Digidiki, V., & Bhabha, J. (2021). Against the best interests of the child: The global injustice of migrant externalization. In L. Weber & C. Tazreiter (Eds.), *Handbook of migration and global justice* (pp. 100–118). Edward Elgar.

Dorsey, M. E., & Díaz-Barriga, M. (2015). The constitution free zone in the United States: Law and life in a state of carcelment. *PoLAR: Political and Legal Anthropology Review*, 38(2), 204–225.

Doty, R. L. (2011). Bare life: Border-crossing deaths and spaces of moral alibi. *Environment and Planning D: Society and Space*, 29(4), 599–612.

Dowling, J. A., & Inda, J. X. (2013). *Governing immigration through crime*. Stanford University Press.

Dreby, J. (2010). *Divided by borders: Mexican migrants and their children*. University of California Press.

Dreby, J. (2012). *How today's immigration enforcement policies impact children, families, and communities: A view from the ground*. Center for American Progress.

Dreby, J. (2015). U.S. immigration policy and family separation: The consequences for children's well-being. *Social Science & Medicine*, 132, 245–251.

Dubal, S. B., Samra, S. S., & Janeway, H. H. (2021). Beyond border health: Infrastructural violence and the health of border abolition. *Social Science & Medicine*, 279, 113967.

Dubos, R. J., & Dubos, J. (1987). *The white plague: Tuberculosis, man, and society*. Rutgers University Press.

Duncan, W. L. (2014). Transnational disorders: Returned migrants at Oaxaca's psychiatric hospital. *Medical Anthropology Quarterly*, 29(1), 24–41.

Durham, J., Brolan, C. E., Lui, C. W., & Whittaker, M. (2016). The need for a rights-based public health approach to Australian asylum seeker health. *Public Health Reviews*, 37(1), 1–24.

Düvell, F. (2006). *Crossing the fringes of Europe: Transit migration in the EU'S neighbourhood*. COMPAS Working Paper. WP-06-33. Centre on Migration, Policy and Society, University of Oxford. www.compas.ox.ac.uk/fileadmin/files/pdfs/WP0633-Duvell.pdf

Düvell, F., & Jordan, B. (2002). Immigration, asylum and welfare: The European context. *Critical Social Policy*, 22(3), 498–517.

Ehrenreich, B., Hochschild, A. R., & Kay, S. (Eds.). (2003). *Global woman: Nannies, maids, and sex workers in the new economy*. Macmillan.

Eichelberger, L. (2007). SARS and Chinatown: The politics of risk and blame during an epidemic of fear. *Social Science & Medicine*, 65(6), 1284–1295.

El Ghazouani, D. (2019). *A growing destination for sub-Saharan Africans, Morocco wrestles with immigrant integration*. Migration Policy Institute. www.migrationpolicy.org/article/ growing-destination-sub-saharan-africans-morocco

Enriquez, L. E. (2015). Multigenerational punishment: Shared experiences of undocumented immigration status within mixed-status families. *Journal of Marriage and Family*, 77(4), 939–953.

Ernst, G. (2000). The myth of the "Mediterranean syndrome": Do immigrants feel different pain? *Ethnicity & Health*, 5(2), 121–126.
Escobar, J. I., & Vega, W. A. (2000). Mental health and immigration's AAAs: Where are we and where do we go from here? *The Journal of Nervous and Mental Disease*, 188(11), 736–740.
Estévez, A. (2012). *Human rights, migration, and social conflict: Towards a decolonized global justice.* Springer.
Fairchild, A. L. (2004). Policies of inclusion: Immigrants, disease, dependency, and American immigration policy at the dawn and dusk of the 20th century. *American Journal of Public Health*, 94(4), 528–539.
Falge, C., & Ruzza, C. (2016). *Migrants and health: Political and institutional responses to cultural diversity in health systems.* Routledge.
Farmer, P. (2001). *Infections and inequalities: The modern plagues.* University of California Press.
Farmer, P. (2003). *Pathologies of power: Health, human rights, and the new war on the poor.* University of California Press.
Fassin, D. (2005). Compassion and repression: The moral economy of immigration policies in France. *Cultural Anthropology*, 20(3), 362–387.
Fassin, D. (2011). Policing borders, producing boundaries. The governmentality of immigration in dark times. *Annual Review of Anthropology*, 40, 213–226.
Fassin, D., & D'Halluin, E. (2005). The truth from the body: Medical certificates as ultimate evidence for asylum seekers. *American Anthropologist*, 107(4), 597–608.
Fennelly, K. (2007). The "healthy migrant" effect. *Minnesota Medicine*, 90(3), 51–53.
Ferhani, A., & Rushton, S. (2020). The international health regulations, COVID-19, and bordering practices: Who gets in, what gets out, and who gets rescued? *Contemporary Security Policy*, 41(3), 458–477.
Fiałkowska, K. (2019). Remote fatherhood and visiting husbands: Seasonal migration and men's position within families. *Comparative Migration Studies*, 7(1), Article 2.
Filc, D., & Davidovich, N. (2005). Health care as a national right? The development of health care services for migrant workers in Israel. *Social Theory & Health*, 3, 1–15.
Fix, M. E., & Tumlin, K. C. (1997). *Welfare reform and the devolution of immigrant policy.* Urban Institute.
Fleischman, Y., Willen, S. S., Davidovitch, N., & Mor, Z. (2015). Migration as a social determinant of health for irregular migrants: Israel as case study. *Social Science & Medicine*, 147, 89–97.
Flores-González, N. (2017). *Citizens but not Americans: Race and belonging among Latino millennials.* New York University Press.
Flynn, M. A. (2018). Im/migration, work, and health: Anthropology and the occupational health of labor im/migrants. *Anthropology of Work Review*, 39(2), 116–123.
Flynn, M. A., Eggerth, D. E., & Jacobson, C. J., Jr. (2015). Undocumented status as a social determinant of occupational safety and health: The workers' perspective. *American Journal of Industrial Medicine*, 58(11), 1127–1137.
Fouron, G., & Schiller, N. G. (2001). All in the family: Gender, transnational migration, and the nation-state. *Identities Global Studies in Culture and Power*, 7(4), 539–582.
Furman, R., Lamphear, G., & Epps, D. (Eds.). (2016). *The immigrant other: Lived experiences in a transnational world.* Columbia University Press.
Galemba, R. B. (2021). "They steal our work": Wage theft and the criminalization of immigrant day laborers in Colorado, U.S.A. *European Journal on Criminal Policy and Research*, 27(1), 91–112.
Gallo, E. (2006). Italy is not a good place for men: Narratives of places, marriage and asculinity among Malayali migrants. *Global Networks*, 6(4), 357–372.

Gamburd, M. R. (2000). *The kitchen spoon's handle: Transnationalism and Sri Lanka's migrant housemaids*. Cornell University Press.

Gamella, J. F. (2018). Marriage, gender and transnational migrations in fertility transitions of Romanian Roma women. *Intersections*, 4(2), 57–85.

Gandy, M., & Zumla, A. (2002). The resurgence of disease: Social and historical perspectives on the "new" tuberculosis. *Social Science & Medicine*, 55(3), 385–396.

Garcia, S. J. (2017). Bridging critical race theory and migration: Moving beyond assimilation theories. *Sociology Compass*, 11(6), e12484.

García Hernández, C. C. (2015). The life of crimmigration law. *Denver University Law Review*, 92(4), 15–46.

Garin, E., Beise J., Hug L., & You, D. (2016). *Uprooted: The growing crisis for refugee and migrant children*. UNICEF. www.unicef.org/publications/files/Uprooted_growing_crisis_for_refugee_and_migrant_children. pdf

Gee, G. C., Walsemann, K. M., & Brondolo, E. (2012). A life course perspective on how racism may be related to health inequities. *American Journal of Public Health*, 102(5), 967–974.

Gideon, J. (2016). Mental health and forced migration: The case of Chilean exiles in the UK. In F. Thomas (Ed.), *Handbook of migration and health* (pp. 318–339). Edward Elgar.

Gielis, R., & van Houtum, H. (2012). Sloterdijk in the house! Dwelling in the borderscape of Germany and The Netherlands. *Geopolitics*, 17(4), 797–817.

Ginsburg, F., & Rapp, R. (1991). The politics of reproduction. *Annual Review of Anthropology*, 20(1), 311–343.

Ginsburg, F., & Rapp, R. (1995). *Conceiving the new world order: The global politics of reproduction*. University of California Press.

Giuntella, O., Kone, Z. L., Ruiz, I., & Vargas-Silva, C. (2018). Reason for immigration and immigrants' health. *Public Health*, 158, 102–109.

Gleeson, S. (2012). Leveraging health capital at the workplace: An examination of health reporting behavior among Latino immigrant restaurant workers in the United States. *Social Science & Medicine*, 75(12), 2291–2298.

Golash-Boza, T. M. (2015). *Deported: Immigrant policing, disposable labor, and global capitalism*. New York University Press.

Golash-Boza, T. M., & Hondagneu-Sotelo, P. (2013). Latino immigrant men and the deportation crisis: A gendered racial removal program. *Latino Studies*, 11(3), 271–292.

Goldade, K. (2009). "Health is hard here" or "health for all"? The politics of blame, gender, and health care for undocumented Nicaraguan migrants in Costa Rica. *Medical Anthropology Quarterly*, 23(4), 483–503.

Goldade, K. (2011). Babies and belonging: Reproduction, citizenship, and undocumented Nicaraguan labor migrant women in Costa Rica. *Medical Anthropology*, 30(5), 545–568.

Goldstein, D. M. (2010). Toward a critical anthropology of security. *Current Anthropology*, 51(4), 487–517.

Gomberg-Munoz, R. (2016). *Becoming legal: Immigration law and mixed-status families*. Oxford University Press.

Gomberg-Munoz, R., & Nussbaum-Barberena, L. (2011). Is immigration policy labor policy? Immigration enforcement, undocumented workers, and the state. *Human Organization*, 70(4), 366–375.

Gonzales, R. G. (2011). Learning to be illegal: Undocumented youth and shifting legal contexts in the transition to adulthood. *American Sociological Review*, 76(4), 602–619.

Gonzales, R. G., Suárez-Orozco, C., & Dedios-Sanguineti, M. C. (2013). No place to belong: Contextualizing concepts of mental health among undocumented immigrant youth in the United States. *American Behavioral Scientist*, 57(8), 1174–1199.

González-López, G. (2005). *Erotic journeys: Mexican immigrants and their sex lives.* University of California Press.

Good, M. J. D., & Good, B. J. (2003). Introduction: Culture in the politics of mental health research. *Culture, Medicine and Psychiatry*, 27(4), 369–371.

Gottlieb, N., Filc, D., & Davidovitch, N. (2012). Medical humanitarianism, human rights and political advocacy: The case of the Israeli open clinic. *Social Science & Medicine*, 74(6), 839–845.

Gottlieb, N., & Schülle, M. (2021). An overview of health policies for asylum-seekers in Germany. *Health Policy*, 125(1), 115–121.

Grabell, M., & Berkes, H. (2015). *The demolition of workers' comp.* ProPublica and National Public Radio.

Grace, B. L., Nawyn, S. J., & Okwako, B. (2018). The right to belong (if you can afford it): Market-based restrictions on social citizenship in refugee resettlement. *Journal of Refugee Studies*, 31(1), 42–62.

Gray, B. (2011). Becoming non-migrant: Lives worth waiting for. *Gender, Place & Culture*, 18(3), 417–432.

Green, L. (2011). The nobodies: neoliberalism, violence, and migration. *Medical anthropology*, 30(4), 366–385.

Groark, C., Sclare, I., & Raval, H. (2011). Understanding the experiences and emotional needs of unaccompanied asylum-seeking adolescents in the UK. *Clinical Child Psychology and Psychiatry*, 16(3), 421–442.

Grove, N. J., & Zwi, A. B. (2006). Our health and theirs: Forced migration, othering, and public health. *Social Science & Medicine*, 62(8), 1931–1942.

Grzywacz, J. G., Quandt, S. A., Chen, H., Isom, S., Kiang, L., Vallejos, Q., & Arcury, T. A. (2010). Depressive symptoms among Latino farmworkers across the agricultural season: Structural and situational influences. *Cultural Diversity and Ethnic Minority Psychology*, 16(3), 335–343.

Gushulak, B. (2007). Healthier on arrival? Further insight into the "healthy immigrant effect". *Cmaj*, 176(10), 1439–1440.

Gushulak, B. D., & MacPherson, D. W. (2000). Health issues associated with the smuggling and trafficking of migrants. *Journal of Immigrant Health*, 2(2), 67–78.

Guzys, D., Kenny, A., Dickson-Swift, V., & Threlkeld, G. (2015). A critical review of population health literacy assessment. *BMC Public Health*, 15(1), 1–7.

Hacker, K., Anies, M., Folb, B. L., & Zallman, L. (2015). Barriers to health care for undocumented immigrants: A literature review. *Risk Management and Healthcare Policy*, 8, 175.

Hacker, K., Chu, J., Arsenault, L., & Marlin, R. P. (2012). Provider's perspectives on the impact of Immigration and Customs Enforcement (ICE) activity on immigrant health. *Journal of Health Care for the Poor and Underserved*, 23(2), 651–665.

Hacker, K., Chu, J., Leung, C., Marra, R., Pirie, A., Brahimi, M., ... Marlin, R. P. (2011). The impact of immigration and customs enforcement on immigrant health: Perceptions of immigrants in Everett, Massachusetts, U.S.A. *Social Science & Medicine*, 73(4), 586–594.

Hagan, J. M., Rodriguez, N., Capps, R., & Kabiri, N. (2003). The effects of recent welfare and immigration reforms on Immigrants' access to health care. *International Migration Review*, 37(2), 444–463.

Hagan, J. M., Rodriguez, N., & Castro, B. (2011). Social effects of mass deportations by the United States government, 2000–10. *Ethnic and Racial Studies*, 34(8), 1374–1391.

Han, B.-C. (2020). The viral emergency and the world tomorrow. *El Pais.*

Handley, M. A., Robles, M., Sanford, E., Collins, N., Seligman, H., Defries, T., ... Grieshop, J. (2013). Navigating changing food environments: Transnational perspectives on dietary behaviours and implications for nutrition counselling. *Global Public Health*, 8(3), 245–257.

Handley, M. A., & Sudhinaraset, M. (2017). The important role of binational studies for migration and health research: A review of U.S.-Mexico binational studies and design considerations for addressing critical issues in migrant health. *International Migration*, 55(5), 75–121.

Harper, I., & Raman, P. (2008). Less than human? Diaspora, disease and the question of citizenship. *International Migration*, 46(5), 3–26.

Hedrick, K., Armstrong, G., Coffey, G., & Borschmann, R. (2020). Self-harm among asylum seekers in Australian onshore immigration detention: How incidence rates vary by held detention type. *BMC Public Health*, 20(1), 1–10.

Heyman, J. (1999). United States surveillance over Mexican lives at the border: Snapshots of an emerging regime. *Human Organization*, 58(4), 430–438.

Heyman, J. McC., Núñez, G. G., & Talavera, V. (2009). Health care access and barriers for unauthorized immigrants in El Paso County, Texas. *Family and Community Health*, 32(1), 4–21.

Himmelgreen, D., Romero Daza, N., Cooper, E., & Martinez, D. (2007). "I don't make the soups anymore": Pre-to post-migration dietary and lifestyle changes among Latinos living in West-Central Florida. *Ecology of Food and Nutrition*, 46(5–6), 427–444.

Hirsch, J. S. (2003). *A courtship after marriage: Sexuality and love in Mexican transnational families*. University of California Press.

Ho, M. J. (2003). Migratory journeys and tuberculosis risk. *Medical Anthropology Quarterly*, 17(4), 442–458.

Hoang, L. A., & Yeoh, B. S. (2011). Breadwinning wives and "left-behind" husbands: Men and masculinities in the Vietnamese transnational family. *Gender & Society*, 25(6), 717–739.

Hodes, M., & Vostanis, P. (2019). Practitioner review: Mental health problems of refugee children and adolescents and their management. *Journal of Child Psychology and Psychiatry*, 60(7), 716–731.

Hoffman, B. (2006). Sympathy and exclusion: Access to health care for undocumented immigrants in the United States. In K. Wailoo, J. Livingston, & P. Guarnaccia (Eds.), *A death retold: Jesica Santillan, the bungled transplant, and the paradoxes of medical citizenship* (pp. 237–254). University of North Carolina Press.

Holmes, S. M. (2007). Oaxacans like to work bent over: The naturalization of social suffering among berry farm workers. *International Migration*, 45(3), 39–68.

Holmes, S. M. (2011). Structural vulnerability and hierarchies of ethnicity and citizenship on the farm. *Medical Anthropology*, 30(4), 425–449.

Holmes, S. M. (2012). The clinical gaze in the practice of migrant health: Mexican migrants in the U.S. *Social Science & Medicine*, 74(6), 873–881.

Holmes, S. M. (2013). *Fresh fruit, broken bodies: Migrant farmworkers in the U.S.* University of California Press.

Holmes, S. M., & Castañeda, H. (2016). Representing the European refugee crisis in Germany and beyond: Deservingness and difference, life and death. *American Ethnologist*, 43(1), 12–24.

Hondagneu-Sotelo, P. (2001). *Domestica: Immigrant workers cleaning and caring in the shadows of affluence*. University of California Press.

Hondagneu-Sotelo, P. (Ed.). (2003). *Gender and U.S. immigration: Contemporary trends*. University of California Press.

Hondagneu-Sotelo, P., & Avila, E. (1997). "I'm here, but I'm there": The meanings of Latina transnational motherhood. *Gender & Society*, 11(5), 548–571.

Horner, P., Sanders, L., Martinez, R., Doering-White, J., Lopez, W., & Delva, J. (2014). 'I put a mask on': The human side of deportation effects on Latino youth. *Journal of Social Welfare and Human Rights*, 2(2), 33–47.

Horton, S. B. (2004). Different subjects: The health care system's participation in the differential construction of the cultural citizenship of Cuban refugees and Mexican immigrants. *Medical Anthropology Quarterly*, 18(4), 472–489.

Horton, S. B. (2014). Medical returns as class transformation: Situating Mexican migrants' medical returns within a framework of transnationalism. *Medical Anthropology*, 32(5), 417–432.

Horton, S. B. (2016). *They leave their kidneys in the fields: Illness, injury, and illegality among U.S. farmworkers*. University of California Press.

Horton, S. B., & Barker, J. C. (2010). Stigmatized biologies: Examining the cumulative effects of oral health disparities for Mexican American farmworker children. *Medical Anthropology Quarterly*, 24(2), 199–219.

Hoyez, A. C., & Thomas, F. (2016). Socio-spatial dimensions of healthcare for newly arrived migrants. In F. Thomas (Ed.), *Handbook of migration and health* (pp. 158–172). Edward Elgar.

Huang, Z. J., Yu, S. M., & Ledsky, R. (2006). Health status and health service access and use among children in U.S. immigrant families. *American Journal of Public Health*, 96(4), 634–640.

Hudson, J. L. (2009). Families with mixed eligibility for public coverage: Navigating Medicaid, CHIP, and Uninsurance. *Health Affairs*, 28(4), w697–w709.

Human Rights Watch. (2016). *Seeking refuge: Unaccompanied children in Sweden*. www.hrw.org/report/2016/06/09/seeking-refuge/unaccompanied-children-sweden2016

Huschke, S. (2014). Performing deservingness: Humanitarian health care provision for migrants in Germany. *Social Science & Medicine*, 120, 352–359.

Hunt, L. M., & De Voogd, K. B. (2005). Clinical myths of the cultural "other": Implications for Latino patient care. *Academic Medicine*, 80(10), 918–924.

Hunt, L. M., Schneider, S., & Comer, B. (2004). Should "acculturation" be a variable in health research? A critical review of research on U.S. Hispanics. *Social Science & Medicine*, 59(5), 973–986.

Hutcheon, E., & Lashewicz, B. (2014). Theorizing resilience: Critiquing and unbounding a marginalizing concept. *Disability & Society*, 29(9), 1383–1397.

Inda, J. X. (2006). *Targeting immigrants: Government, technology, and ethics*. Wiley.

Inda, J. X., & Dowling, J. (2013). Introduction: governing migrant illegality. In J. A. Dowling & J. X. Inda (Eds.). *Governing immigration through crime: A reader* (pp. 1–36). Stanford University Press.

International Organization for Migration. (2019). *Glossary on migration*. https://publications.iom.int/system/files/pdf/iml_34_glossary.pdf

International Organization for Migration. (2022). *World migration report 2022*. https://worldmigrationreport.iom.int/wmr-2022-interactive/

Iselin, B., & Adams, M. (2003). Distinguishing between human trafficking and people smuggling. *UN Office on Drugs and Crime*, 1–10. www.embraceni.org/wp-content/uploads/2006/06/Distinguishing[1]1.pdf

Jackson, T. (2003). Mystery of the imported plagues. *BMJ*, 326(7384), 342.

Jacobsen, C. M., Karlsen, M. A., & Khosravi, S. (2021). *Waiting and the temporalities of irregular migration*. Taylor & Francis.

Jass, G., & Massey, D. S. (2004). *Immigrant health: Selectivity and acculturation* (No. 04/23). IFS Working Papers.

Jayaweera, H. (2016). Migration and health behaviour. In F. Thomas (Ed.), *Handbook of migration and health* (pp. 59–74). Edward Elgar.

Jaye, C., & Fitzgerald, R. (2010). The lived political economy of occupational overuse syndrome among New Zealand workers. *Sociology of Health & Illness*, 32(7), 1010–1025.

Jaye, C., & Fitzgerald, R. (2012). The embodied liminalities of occupational overuse syndrome. *Medical Anthropology Quarterly*, 26(2), 201–220.

Jensen, B., Giorguli Saucedo, S., & Hernández Padilla, E. (2016). International migration and the academic performance of Mexican adolescents. *International Migration Review*, 52(2), 559–596.

Joffe, H., & Haarhoff, G. (2002). Representations of far-flung illnesses: The case of Ebola in Britain. *Social Science & Medicine*, 54(6), 955–969.

Johnson, C., Jones, R., Paasi, A., Amoore, L., Mountz, A., Salter, M., & Rumford, C. (2011). Interventions on rethinking "the border" in border studies. *Political Geography*, 30(2), 61–69.

Joseph, T. D., & Marrow, H. B. (2017). Health care, immigrants, and minorities: lessons from the affordable care act in the U.S. *Journal of Ethnic and Migration Studies*, 43(12), 1965–1984.

Jossen, M. (2018). *Undocumented migrants and healthcare: Eight stories from Switzerland.* OpenBook Publishers.

Kaiser, B. N., Keys, H. M., Foster, J., & Kohrt, B. A. (2015). Social stressors, social support, and mental health among Haitian migrants in the Dominican Republic. *Revista Panamericana de Salud Pública*, 38, 157–162.

Karliner, L. S., Jacobs, E. A., Chen, A. H., & Mutha, S. (2007). Do professional interpreters improve clinical care for patients with limited English proficiency? A systematic review of the literature. *Health Services Research*, 42(2), 727–754.

Karlsen, M. A. (2016). Migration control and children's access to healthcare. In F. Thomas (Ed.), *Handbook of migration and health* (pp. 134–157). Edward Elgar.

Kawachi, I., Subramanian, S.V., & Almeida-Filho, N. (2002). A glossary for health inequalities. *Journal of Epidemiology & Community Health*, 56(9), 647–652.

Keller, A. S., Ford, D., Sachs, E., Rosenfeld, B., Trinh-Shevrin, C., Meserve, C., ... Rockline, P. (2003). The impact of detention on the health of asylum seekers. *The Journal of Ambulatory Care Management*, 26(4), 383–385.

Kerwin, D. (2012). The faltering U.S. refugee protection system: Legal and policy responses to refugees, asylum-seekers, and others in need of protection. *Refugee Survey Quarterly*, 31(1), 1–3.

Keygnaert, I., Vettenburg, N., Roelens, K., & Temmerman, M. (2014). Sexual health is dead in my body: Participatory assessment of sexual health determinants by refugees, asylum seekers and undocumented migrants in Belgium and the Netherlands. *BMC Public Health*, 14(1), 1–13.

Khan, L. K., Sobal, J., & Martorell, R. (1997). Acculturation, socioeconomic status, and obesity in Mexican Americans, Cuban Americans, and Puerto Ricans. *International Journal of Obesity*, 21(2), 91–96.

Khan, M. S., Osei-Kofi, A., Omar, A., Kirkbride, H., Kessel, A., Abbara, A., ... Dar, O. (2016). Pathogens, prejudice, and politics: The role of the global health community in the European refugee crisis. *The Lancet Infectious Diseases*, 16(8), e173–e177.

Khosravi, S. (2010). An ethnography of migrant "illegality" in Sweden: Included yet excepted? *Journal of International Political Theory*, 6(1), 95–116.

Kim, D., Subramanian, S. V., & Kawachi, I. (2008). Social capital and physical health. In I. Kawachi, S. V. Subramanian, & D. Kim (Eds.), *Social capital and health* (pp. 139–190). Springer.

Kistemann, T., Munzinger, A., & Dangendorf, F. (2002). Spatial patterns of tuberculosis incidence in Cologne (Germany). *Social Science & Medicine*, 55(1), 7–19.

Kleinman, A. (1980). *Patients and healers in the context of culture.* University of California Press.

Kleinman, A., & Benson, P. (2006). Anthropology in the clinic: The problem of cultural competency and how to fix it. *PLoS Medicine*, 3(10), e294.

Kline, N. (2019). *Pathogenic policing: Immigration enforcement and health in the U.S. South*. Rutgers University Press.

Kline, N. (2020). Rethinking COVID-19 vulnerability: A call for LGBTQ+ im/migrant health equity in the United States during and after a pandemic. *Health Equity*, 4(1), 239–242.

Kline, N., & Castañeda, H. (2019). Immigration enforcement policies and Latinx health: State of knowledge. In A. D. Martinez & S. D. Rhodes (Eds.), *New and emerging issues in Latinx health* (pp. 253–269). Springer International.

Knipper, M. I. (2013). Joining ethnography and history in cultural competence training. *Culture, Medicine, and Psychiatry*, 37(2), 373–384.

Knoll, A., & Teevan, C. (2020). *Protecting migrants and refugees in North Africa: Challenges and opportunities for reform*. https://ecdpm.org/wp-content/uploads/Protecting-Migrants-Refugees-North-Africa-Challenges-Opportunities-Reform-Discussion-Paper-281-October-2020-ECDPM.pdf

Kohli, A., Markowitz, P. L., & Chavez, L. (2011). *Secure communities by the numbers: An analysis of demographics and due process*. Warren Institute of Law and Policy.

Krieger, N. (2013). *Epidemiology and the people's health: Theory and context*. Oxford University Press.

Krieger, N. (2016). *Embodying inequality: Epidemiologic perspectives*. Routledge Press.

Kwon, J. H. (2015). The work of waiting: Love and money in Korean Chinese transnational migration. *Cultural Anthropology*, 30(3), 477–500.

Landolt, P., & Goldring, L. (2016). Assembling noncitizenship through the work of conditionality. *Citizenship Studies*, 19(8), 853–869.

Lara, M., Gamboa, C., Kahramanian, M. I., Morales, L. S., & Hayes Bautista, D. E. (2005). Acculturation and Latino health in the United States: A review of the literature and its sociopolitical context. *Annual Review of Public Health*, 26, 367–397.

Larchanché, S. (2012). Intangible obstacles: Health implications of stigmatization, structural violence, and fear among undocumented immigrants in France. *Social Science & Medicine*, 74(6), 858–863.

Laubenthal, B. (2008). *Two steps forward, one step back: Recent trends in German migration policy*. CeSPI Country paper.

Lawlor, A., & Tolley, E. (2017). Deciding who's legitimate: News media framing of immigrants and refugees. *International Journal of Communication*, 11, 25.

Lee, A., Sim, F., & Mackie, P. (2018). Migration and health: Seeing past the hype, hysteria and labels. *Public Health*, 158, A1–A2.

Lee, J.Y., Kearns, R.A., & Friesen, W. (2010). Seeking affective health care: Korean immigrants' use of homeland medical services. *Health & Place*, 16(1), 108–115.

Lee, S. H. (2021). *Korean wild geese families: Gender, family, social, and legal dynamics of middle-class Asian transnational families in North America*. Lexington Books.

Leigh, J. P., & Robbins, J. A. (2004). Occupational disease and workers' compensation: Coverage, costs, and consequences. *The Milbank Quarterly*, 82(4), 689–721.

Leischow, S. J., & Milstein, B. (2006). Systems thinking and modeling for public health practice. *American Journal of Public Health*, 96(3), 403–405.

Link, B. G., & Phelan, J. (1995). Social conditions as fundamental causes of disease. *Journal of Health and Social Behavior*, (Extra issue), 80–94.

Lippel, K. (2012). Preserving workers' dignity in workers' compensation systems: An international perspective. *American Journal of Industrial Medicine*, 55(6), 519–536.

Lipsky, M. (1980). *Street-level bureaucracy: Dilemmas of the individual in public services*. Russel Sage.

Liu, X., & Bennett, M. M. (2020). Viral borders: COVID-19's effects on securitization, surveillance, and identity in Mainland China and Hong Kong. *Dialogues in Human Geography*, 10(2), 158–163.

Lock, M. M., & Nguyen, V. K. (2018). *An anthropology of biomedicine*. Wiley.
Logan, R. I., Melo, M. A., & Castañeda, H. (2021). Familial vulnerability: Legal status and mental health within mixed-status families. *Medical Anthropology*, 40(7): 639–652.
Logan, R. I. (2022). *Boundaries of Care: Community Health Workers in the United States*. Rowman and Littlefield.
López, L. (2005). De facto disentitlement in an information economy: Enrollment issues in Medicaid managed care. *Medical Anthropology Quarterly*, 19(1), 26–46.
Lopez, M. H., & Minushkin, S., (2008). *National survey of Latinos*. Pew Hispanic Center. http://pewhispanic.org/reports/report.php?ReportID¼93
Lopez, W. D., Kruger, D. J., Delva, J., Llanes, M., Ledón, C., Waller, A., … Harner, M. (2017). Health implications of an immigration raid: Findings from a Latino community in the midwestern U.S. *Journal of Immigrant and Minority Health*, 19(3), 702–708.
Lori, J. R., & Boyle, J. S. (2015). Forced migration: Health and human rights issues among refugee populations. *Nursing Outlook*, 63(1), 68–76.
Lu, Y., & Zhang, A. T. (2016). The link between migration and health. In F. Thomas (Ed.), *Handbook of migration and health* (pp. 19–43). Edward Elgar.
Luibhéid, E. (2002). *Entry denied: Controlling sexuality at the border*. University of Minnesota Press.
Luibhéid, E. (2008). Sexuality, migration, and the shifting line between legal and illegal status. *GLQ: A Journal of Lesbian and Gay Studies*, 14(2–3), 289–315.
Luke, D. A., & Stamatakis, K. A. (2012). Systems science methods in public health: Dynamics, networks, and agents. *Annual Review of Public Health*, 33, 357–376.
Lupton, D. (1999). *Risk*. Routledge Press.
Lupton, D. (2000). *Risk and sociocultural theory: New directions and perspectives*. Cambridge University Press.
Lurie, M. N. (2006). The epidemiology of migration and HIV/AIDS in South Africa. *Journal of Ethnic and Migration Studies*, 32(4), 649–666.
Lurie, M. N., Williams, B. G., Zuma, K., Mkaya-Mwamburi, D., Garnett, G. P., Sturm, A. W., … Karim, S. S. A. (2003). The impact of migration on HIV-1 transmission in South Africa: A study of migrant and nonmigrant men and their partners. *Sexually Transmitted Diseases*, 30(2), 149–156.
Lykes, M. B., Brabeck, K. M., & Hunter, C. J. (2013). Exploring parent–child communication in the context of threat: Immigrant families facing detention and deportation in post-9/11 U.S.A. *Community, Work & Family*, 16(2), 123–146.
Lysakowski, M., Persall, A., & Pope, J. (2016). *Policing in new immigrant communities*. U.S. Department of Justice.
MacEachen, E. (2000). The mundane administration of worker bodies: From welfarism to neoliberalism. *Health, Risk & Society*, 2(3), 315–327.
MacFarlane, A., Dzebisova, Z., Karapish, D., Kovacevic, B., Ogbebor, F., & Okonkwo, E. (2009). Arranging and negotiating the use of informal interpreters in general practice consultations: Experiences of refugees and asylum seekers in the west of Ireland. *Social Science & Medicine*, 69(2), 210–214.
Magalhaes, L., Carrasco, C., & Gastaldo, D. (2010). Undocumented migrants in Canada: A scope literature review on health, access to services, and working conditions. *Journal of Immigrant and Minority Health*, 12(1), 132–151.
Mainwaring, Ċ., & Brigden, N. (2016). Beyond the border: Clandestine migration journeys. *Geopolitics*, 21(2), 243–262.
Makariev, D. W., & Shaver, P. R. (2010). Attachment, parental incarceration and possibilities for intervention: An overview. *Attachment & Human Development*, 12(4), 311–331.

Maldonado, C. Z., Rodriguez, R. M., Torres, J. R., Flores, Y. S., & Lovato, L. M. (2013). Fear of discovery among Latino immigrants presenting to the emergency department. *Academic Emergency Medicine*, 20(2), 155–161.

Malkki, L. H. (1995). Refugees and exile: From "refugee studies" to the national order of things. *Annual Review of Anthropology*, 24(1), 495–523.

Malkki, L. H. (1996). Speechless emissaries: Refugees, humanitarianism, and dehistoricization. *Cultural Anthropology*, 11(3), 377–404.

Manalansan, M. F., IV. (2006). Queer intersections: Sexuality and gender in migration studies. *International Migration Review*, 40(1), 224–249.

Manderson, L., & Allotey, P. (2003). Storytelling, marginality, and community in Australia: How immigrants position their difference in health care settings. *Medical Anthropology*, 22(1), 1–21.

Manderson, L., & Smith-Morris, C. (2010). Introduction: Chronicity and the experience of illness. In L. Manderson & C. Smith-Morris (Eds.), *Chronic conditions, fluid states* (pp. 1–18). Rutgers University Press.

Marciniak, K. (2006). *Alienhood: Citizenship, exile, and the logic of difference*. University of Minnesota Press.

Marín, A., Carrillo, L., Arcury, T. A., Grzywacz, J. G., Coates, M. L., & Quandt, S. A. (2009). Ethnographic evaluation of a lay health promoter program to reduce occupational injuries among Latino poultry processing workers. *Public Health Reports*, 124(4 Suppl. 1), 36–43.

Marrow, H. (2011). *New destination dreaming: Immigration, race, and legal status in the rural American South*. Stanford University Press.

Marrow, H. B. (2012). Deserving to a point: Unauthorized immigrants in San Francisco's universal access healthcare model. *Social Science & Medicine*, 74(6), 846–854.

Mason-Jones, A. J., & Nicholson, P. (2018). Structural violence and marginalisation. The sexual and reproductive health experiences of separated young people on the move. A rapid review with relevance to the European humanitarian crisis. *Public Health*, 158, 156–162.

Massey, D. S. (2020). Immigration policy mismatches and counterproductive outcomes: Unauthorized migration to the U.S. in two eras. *Comparative Migration Studies*, 8(1), 1–27.

Mata-Codesal, D. (2015). Ways of staying put in Ecuador: Social and embodied experiences of mobility–immobility interactions. *Journal of Ethnic and Migration Studies*, 41(14), 2274–2290.

Mbembé, J.-A. (2003). Necropolitics. *Public Culture*, 15(1), 11–40.

McCoy, C. (2020). *Diseased states: Epidemic control in Britain and the U.S.* University of Massachusetts Press.

McElrone, M., Colby, S. E., Moret, L., Kavanagh, K., Spence, M., Fouts, H. N., … Payne, M. (2019). Barriers and facilitators to food security among adult Burundian and Congolese refugee females resettled in the U.S. *Ecology of Food and Nutrition*, 58(3), 247–264.

McGuire, S., Sr., & Georges, J. (2003). Undocumentedness and liminality as health variables. *Advances in Nursing Science*, 26(3), 185–195.

McKenzie, D., & Rapoport, H. (2006). *Can migration reduce educational attainment? Evidence from Mexico* (Policy Research Working Paper No. 3952). World Bank.

McLeigh, J. D. (2010). How do immigration and customs enforcement (ICE) practices affect the mental health of children? *American Journal of Orthopsychiatry*, 80(1), 96–100.

McMahon, S., & Sigona, N. (2021). Death and migration: Migrant journeys and the governance of migration during Europe's "Migration Crisis." *International Migration Review*, 55(2), 605–628.

McMichael, C. (2020). Human mobility, climate change, and health: Unpacking the connections. *The Lancet Planetary Health*, 4(6), e217–e218.

McNeill, P. M. (2003). Public health ethics: Asylum seekers and the case for political action. *Bioethics*, 17(5–6), 487–503.

McSwiggin, C. (2017). Moral adherence: HIV treatment, undetectability, and stigmatized viral loads among Haitians in South Florida. *Medical Anthropology*, 36(8), 714–728.

Mekouaz, H. (2020) The hardship of foreign migrants in Morocco. *The North Africa Journal*. https://north-africa.com/2020/05/morocco-the-hardship-of-foreign-migrants-in-morocco/

Mels, C., Derluyn, I., Broekaert, E., & Rosseel, Y. (2010). The psychological impact of forced displacement and related risk factors on Eastern Congolese adolescents affected by war. *Journal of Child Psychology and Psychiatry*, 51(10), 1096–1104.

Mendenhall, E. (2016). Beyond comorbidity: A critical perspective of syndemic depression and diabetes in cross-cultural contexts. *Medical Anthropology Quarterly*, 30(4), 462–478.

Mendenhall, E., Kohrt, B. A., Norris, S. A., Ndetei, D., & Prabhakaran, D. (2017). Non-communicable disease syndemics: Poverty, depression, and diabetes among low-income populations. *Lancet*, 389(10072), 951–963.

Mendoza, F. S. (2009). Health disparities and children in immigrant families: A research agenda. *Pediatrics*, 124(Suppl. 3), S187–S195.

Menjívar, C. (2011). The power of the law: Central Americans' legality and everyday life in Phoenix, Arizona. *Latino Studies*, 9(4), 377–395.

Menjívar, C. (2014). Immigration law beyond borders: Externalizing and internalizing border controls in an era of securitization. *Annual Review of Law and Social Science*, 10, 353–369.

Menjívar, C., & Abrego, L. J. (2009). Parents and children across Borders: Legal instability and intergenerational relations in Guatemalan and Salvadoran Families. In N. Foner (Ed.), *Across generations: Immigrant families in America* (pp. 160–189). NYU Press.

Menjívar, C., & Abrego, L. J. (2012). Legal violence: Immigration law and the lives of Central American immigrants. *American Journal of Sociology*, 117(5), 1380–1421.

Menjívar, C., Abrego, L. J., & Schmalzbauer, L. C. (2016). *Immigrant families*. Wiley.

Menjívar, C., & Agadjanian, V. (2007). Men's migration and women's lives: Views from rural Armenia and Guatemala. *Social Science Quarterly*, 88(5), 1243–1262.

Menjívar, C., & Kanstroom, D. (Eds.). (2013). *Constructing immigrant "illegality": Critiques, experiences, and responses*. Cambridge University Press.

Metzl, J. M., & Hansen, H. (2014). Structural competency: Theorizing a new medical engagement with stigma and inequality. *Social Science & Medicine*, 103, 126–133.

Meuter, R. F., Gallois, C., Segalowitz, N. S., Ryder, A. G., & Hocking, J. (2015). Overcoming language barriers in healthcare: A protocol for investigating safe and effective communication when patients or clinicians use a second language. *BMC Health Services Research*, 15(1), 1–5.

Minn, P. (2010). Medical humanitarianism and health as a human right on the Haitian-Dominican border. P. Zacair (Ed.), *Haiti and the Haitian diaspora in the wider Caribbean* (pp. 103–120). University Press of Florida.

Miranda, J., & Legha, R. (2019). The consequences of family separation at the border and beyond. *Journal of the American Academy of Child and Adolescent Psychiatry*, 58(1), 139–140.

Missbach, A. (2015). *Troubled transit: Asylum seekers stuck in Indonesia*. ISEAS-Yusof Ishak Institute.

Mladovsky, P., Ingleby, D., & Rechel, B. (2012). Good practices in migrant health: The European experience. *Clinical Medicine*, 12(3), 248–252.

Monaghan, P. (2011). Lessons learned from a community coalition with diverse stakeholders: The partnership for citrus worker health. *Annals of Anthropological Practice*, 35(2), 27–42.

Montoya, M. J. (2007). Bioethnic conscription: Genes, race, and Mexicana/o ethnicity in diabetes research. *Cultural Anthropology*, 22(1), 94–128.

Morof, D. F., Sami, S., Mangeni, M., Blanton, C., Cardozo, B. L., & Tomczyk, B. (2014). A cross-sectional survey on gender-based violence and mental health among female urban refugees and asylum seekers in Kampala, Uganda. *International Journal of Gynecology & Obstetrics*, 127(2), 138–143.

Mourji, F., Ferrié, J. N., Radi, S., & Alioua, M. (2016). Les migrants subsahariens au Maroc. Enjeux d̕une migration de résidence. Konrad Adenauer Stiftung. www.kas.de/c/document_library/get_file?uuid=5757725d-390b-3cbf-1151-999a9653f572&groupId=252038

Neff, J., Knight, K. R., Satterwhite, S., Nelson, N., Matthews, J., & Holmes, S. M. (2017). Teaching structure: A qualitative evaluation of a structural competency training for resident physicians. *Journal of General Internal Medicine*, 32(4), 430–433.

Nevins, J. (2001). *Operation gatekeeper: The rise of the "illegal alien" and the remaking of the U.S.–Mexico boundary*. Routledge.

Ngai, M. (2014). *Impossible subjects: Illegal aliens and the making of modern America*. Princeton University Press.

Nielsen-Bohlman, L., Panzer, A. M., & Kindig, D. A. (Eds.). (2004). *Health literacy: A prescription to end confusion*. National Academies Press.

Okeke-Ihejirika, P., Yohani, S., Muster, J., Ndem, A., Chambers, T., & Pow, V. (2020). A scoping review on intimate partner violence in Canada's immigrant communities. *Trauma, Violence, & Abuse*, 21(4), 788–810.

Olwig, K. F. (1999). Narratives of the children left behind: Home and identity in globalised Caribbean families. *Journal of Ethnic and Migration Studies*, 25(2), 267–284.

Oztig, L. I. (2016). Justification by the U.S. and India for their border controls against illegal immigration. *Asian Journal of Political Science*, 24(3), 269–284.

Padilla, M. (2007). *Caribbean pleasure industry: Tourism, sexuality, and AIDS in the Dominican Republic. Worlds of desire*. The University of Chicago Press.

Park, L. S. H. (2011). Criminalizing immigrant mothers: Public charge, health care, and welfare reform. *International Journal of Sociology of the Family*, 37(1), 27–47.

Parker, N., & Vaughan-Williams, N. (2009). Lines in the sand? Towards an agenda for critical border studies. *Geopolitics*, 14(3), 582–587.

Parker, N., & Vaughan-Williams, N. (2012). Critical border studies: Broadening and deepening the "lines in the sand" agenda. *Geopolitics*, 17(4), 727–733.

Parrenas, R. S. (2001). *Servants of globalization: Women, migration and domestic work*. Stanford University Press.

Pauli, J. (2008). A house of one's own: Gender, migration, and residence in rural Mexico. *American Ethnologist*, 35 (1), 171–187.

Pavlish, C. L., Noor, S., & Brandt, J. (2010). Somali immigrant women and the American health care system: Discordant beliefs, divergent expectations, and silent worries. *Social Science & Medicine*, 71(2), 353–361.

Peckham, T. K., Baker, M. G., Camp, J. E., Kaufman, J. D., & Seixas, N. S. (2017). Creating a future for occupational health. *Annals of Work Exposures and Health*, 61(1), 3–15.

Perreira, K. M., Crosnoe, R., Fortuny, K., Pedroza, J., Ulvestad, K., Weiland, C., … Chaudry, A. (2012). *Barriers to immigrants' access to health and human services programs*. ASPE Issue Brief. Office of the Assistant Secretary for Planning and Evaluation.

Pessar, P. R., & Mahler, S. J. (2003). Transnational migration: Bringing gender in. *International Migration Review*, 37(3), 812–846.

Peutz, N., & De Genova, N. (2010). *The deportation regime: Sovereignty, space, and the freedom of movement*. Duke University Press.

Phelan, J. C., & Link, B. G. (2015). Is racism a fundamental cause of inequalities in health? *Annual Review of Sociology*, 41, 311–330.
Phelan, J. C., Link, B. G., & Tehranifar, P. (2010). Social conditions as fundamental causes of health inequalities: Theory, evidence, and policy implications. *Journal of Health and Social Behavior*, 51(1 Suppl.), S28–S40.
Phillips, M., & Missbach, A. (2017). Introduction to the special issue on transit migration: Renewing the focus on a global phenomenon. *International Journal of Migration and Border Studies*, 3(2), 113–120.
Phillips, S., Hagan, J. M., & Rodriguez, N. (2006). Brutal borders? Examining the treatment of deportees during arrest and detention. *Social Forces*, 85(1), 93–109.
Pickwell, S. (1999). Multilevel healing pursuits of Cambodian refugees. *Journal of Immigrant Health*, 1(3), 165–179.
Poduval, S., Howard, N., Jones, L., Murwill, P., McKee, M., & Legido-Quigley, H. (2015). Experiences among undocumented migrants accessing primary care in the United Kingdom: A qualitative study. *International Journal of Health Services*, 45(2), 320–333.
Poeze, M., & Mazzucato, V. (2013). Ghanaian children in transnational families: Understanding the experiences of left-behind children through local parenting norms. In L. Baldassar & L. Merla (Eds.), *Transnational families, migration and the circulation of care* (pp. 165–185). Routledge.
Portes, A., & Rumbaut, R. (2001). *Legacies: The story of the immigrant second generation*. University of California Press.
Poss, J., & Jezewski, M. A. (2002). The role and meaning of susto in Mexican Americans' explanatory model of type 2 diabetes. *Medical Anthropology Quarterly*, 16(3), 360–377.
Pransky, G., Moshenberg, D., Benjamin, K., Portillo, S., Thackrey, J. L., & Hill-Fotouhi, C. (2002). Occupational risks and injuries in non-agricultural immigrant Latino workers. *American Journal of Industrial Medicine*, 42(2), 117–123.
Premkumar, A., Raad, K., & Haidar, M. H. (2016). Rethinking the social history in the era of biolegitimacy: Global health and medical education in the care of Palestinian and Syrian refugees in Beirut, Lebanon. *Anthropology & Medicine*, 23(1), 14–29.
Quandt, S. A., Hernández-Valero, M. A., Grzywacz, J. G., Hovey, J. D., Gonzales, M., & Arcury, T. A. (2006). Workplace, household, and personal predictors of pesticide exposure for farmworkers. *Environmental Health Perspectives*, 114(6), 943–952.
Quesada, J., Hart, L. K., & Philippe, B. (2011). Structural vulnerability and health: Latino migrant laborers in the U.S. *Medical Anthropology*, 30(4), 339–362.
Rabin, N. (2009). *Unseen prisoners: A report on women in immigration detention facilities in Arizona. Georgetown Immigration Law Review*, 23(4), 695–763.
Redclift, V. (2013a). Abjects or agents? Camps, contests, and the creation of "political space." *Citizenship Studies*, 17(3–4), 308–321.
Redclift, V. (2013b). *Statelessness and citizenship: Camps and the creation of political space*. Routledge.
Reich, A. D., Hansen, H. B., & Link, B. G. (2016). Fundamental interventions: How clinicians can address the fundamental causes of disease. *Journal of Bioethical Inquiry*, 13(2), 185–192.
Rhodes, S. D., Mann, L., Simán, F. M., Song, E., Alonzo, J., Downs, M., … Hall, M. A. (2015). The impact of local immigration enforcement policies on the health of immigrant Hispanics/Latinos in the United States. *American Journal of Public Health*, 105(2), 329–337.
Robertson, A. M., Lozada, R., Vera, A., Palinkas, L. A., Burgos, J. L., Magis-Rodriguez, C., … Ojeda, V. D. (2012). Deportation experiences of women who inject drugs in Tijuana, Mexico. *Qualitative Health Research*, 22(4), 499–510.
Rodgers, D., & O'Neill, B. (2012). Infrastructural violence: Introduction to the special issue. *Ethnography*, 13(4), 401–412.

Rodriguez, N. G. L. (2017). *Fragile families*. University of Pennsylvania Press.
Romero-Ortuño, R. (2004). Access to health care for illegal immigrants in the EU: Should we be concerned. *European Journal of Health Law*, 11, 245–272.
Rosas, G. (2006). The managed violences of the borderlands: Treacherous geographies, policeability, and the politics of race. *Latino Studies*, 4(4), 401–418.
Rosenthal, A. (2007). Illegality and illness in the everyday struggles of undocumented HIV+ migrant workers in Tel Aviv. *International Migration*, 45(3), 134–156.
Roura, M., Bisoffi, F., Navaza, B., & Pool, R. (2015). "Carrying Ibuprofen in the bag": Priority health concerns of Latin American migrants in Spain – a participatory qualitative study. *PLoS One*, 10(8), e0136315.
Ruef, A. M., Litz, B. T., & Schlenger, W. E. (2000). Hispanic ethnicity and risk for combat-related posttraumatic stress disorder. *Cultural Diversity and Ethnic Minority Psychology*, 6(3), 235–251.
Rutter, M. (1979). Maternal deprivation, 1972-1978: New findings, new concepts, new approaches. *Child Development* , 50(2), 283–305.
Salas, L. M., Ayón, C., & Gurrola, M. (2013). Estamos traumados: The effect of anti-immigrant sentiment and policies on the mental health of Mexican immigrant families. *Journal of Community Psychology*, 41(8), 1005–1020.
Samari, G. (2016). Cross-border ties and Arab American mental health. *Social Science & Medicine*, 155, 93–101.
Sargent, C. (2006). Reproductive strategies and Islamic discourse: Malian migrants negotiate everyday life in Paris, France. *Medical Anthropology Quarterly*, 20(1), 31–49.
Sargent, C. (2012). "Deservingness" and the politics of healthcare. *Social Science & Medicine*, 74, 855–857.
Saunders, S. L., & Nedelec, B. (2014). What work means to people with work disability: A scoping review. *Journal of Occupational Rehabilitation*, 24(1), 100–110.
Saxton, D. I., & Stuesse, A. (2018). Workers' decompensation: Engaged research with injured im/migrant workers. *Anthropology of Work Review*, 39(2), 65–78.
Schapendonk, J. (2007). Staying put in moving sands: The stepwise migration process of sub-Saharan African migrants heading North. *Respacing Africa*, 4, 113–138.
Schapendonk, J. (2012). Migrants' im/mobilities on their way to the EU: Lost in transit?" *Tijdschrift voor economische en sociale geografie*, 103(4), 577–583.
Schapendonk, J. (2013). Sub-Saharan migrants heading north: A mobility perspective. *Africa-Europe Group for Interdisciplinary Studies*, 8, 9–23.
Schenker, M. B. (2010). A global perspective of migration and occupational health. *American Journal of Industrial Medicine*, 53(4), 329–337.
Schierup, C. U., & Jørgensen, M. B. (2017). From "social exclusion" to "precarity." The becoming-migrant of labour: An introduction. In M. B. Jørgensen & C. U. Schierup (Eds.), *Politics of precarity* (pp. 1–29). Brill.
Schouten, B. C., & Schinkel, S. (2014). Turkish migrant GP patients' expression of emotional cues and concerns in encounters with and without informal interpreters. *Patient Education and Counseling*, 97(1), 23–29.
Segura, D. A., & Zavella, P. (Eds.). (2007). *Women and migration in the U.S.-Mexico borderlands: A reader*. Duke University Press.
Sheller, M., & Urry, J. (2006). The new mobilities paradigm. *Environment and Planning A*, 38(2), 207–226.
Shonkoff, J. P., Boyce, W. T., & McEwen, B. S. (2009). Neuroscience, molecular biology, and the childhood roots of health disparities: Building a new framework for health promotion and disease prevention. *JAMA*, 301(21), 2252–2259.
Sigona, N. (2012). I've too much baggage: The impact of *legal* status on the social worlds of irregular migrants. *Social Anthropology/Anthropologie Sociale*, 20(1), 50–65.

Sigvardsdotter, E., Malm, A., Tinghög, P., Vaez, M., & Saboonchi, F. (2016). Refugee trauma measurement: A review of existing checklists. *Public Health Reviews*, 37(1), 1–9.
Sime, D. (2016). Migrant children and young people's "voice" in healthcare. In F. Thomas (Ed.), *Handbook of migration and health*. (pp. 419–437). Edward Elgar.
Singer, M. (2000). A dose of drugs, a touch of violence, a case of AIDS: Conceptualizing the SAVA syndemic. *Free Inquiry in Creative Sociology*, 28(1), 13–24.
Singer, M., & Clair, S. (2003). Syndemics and public health: Reconceptualizing disease in bio-social context. *Medical Anthropology Quarterly*, 17(4), 423–441.
Singer, M., & Rylko-Bauer, B. (2021). Syndemics and structural violence of the COVID pandemic: Anthropological insights on a crisis. *Open Anthropological Research*, 1(1), 7–32.
Sládková, J., Mangado, S. M. G., & Quinteros, J. R. (2012). Lowell immigrant communities in the climate of deportations. *Analyses of Social Issues and Public Policy* (ASAP), 12(1), 78–95.
Smith, C. J., & Yang, X. (2005). Examining the connection between temporary migration and the spread of STDs and HIV/AIDS in China. *China Review*, 5(1), 111–139.
Smith-Nonini, S. (2011). The illegal and the dead: Are Mexicans renewable energy? *Medical Anthropology*, 30(5), 454–474.
Sommers, B. D., Tomasi, M. R., Swartz, K., & Epstein, A. M. (2012). Reasons for the wide variation in Medicaid participation rates among states hold lessons for coverage expansion in 2014. *Health Affairs*, 31(5), 909–919.
Sousa, E., Agudelo-Suárez, A., Benavides, F. G., Schenker, M., García, A. M., Benach, J., … Porthé, V. (2010). Immigration, work and health in Spain: The influence of legal status and employment contract on reported health indicators. *International Journal of Public Health*, 55(5), 443–451.
Spallek, J., Reeske, A., Zeeb, H., & Razum, O. (2016). Models of migration and health. In F. Thomas (Ed.), *Handbook of migration and health* (pp. 44–58). Edward Elgar.
Spiegel, P. B. (2004). HIV/AIDS among conflict-affected and displaced populations: Dispelling myths and taking action. *Disasters*, 28(3), 322–339.
Spiegel, P. B., Bennedsen, A. R., Claass, J., Bruns, L., Patterson, N., Yiweza, D., & Schilperoord, M. (2007). Prevalence of HIV infection in conflict-affected and displaced people in seven sub-Saharan African countries: A systematic review. *The Lancet*, 369(9580), 2187–2195.
Spitzer, D. L. (2016). Migration and health through an intersectional lens. In F. Thomas (Ed.), *Handbook of migration and health* (pp. 75–94). Edward Elgar.
Srikantiah, J. (2007). Perfect victims and real survivors: The iconic victim in domestic human trafficking law. *Boston University Law Review*, 87, 157–212.
Sterling-Folker, J., Freyberg-Inan, A., Wilcox, L., Ozguc, U., & Shinko, R. E. (2021). Thinking theoretically in unsettled times: COVID-19 and beyond. *International Studies Review*, 23(3), 1100–1125.
Stock, I. (2012). Gender and dynamics of mobility: Reflections on African migrant mothers and "Transit Migration" in Morocco. *Ethnic and Racial Studies*, 35(9), 1577–1595.
Stock, I. (2019). *Time, migration and forced immobility: Sub-Saharan African migrants in Morocco*. Bristol University Press.
Stone, S. D. (2003). Workers without work: Injured workers and well-being. *Journal of Occupational Science*, 10(1), 7–13.
Stonington, S. D., Holmes, S. M., Hansen, H., Greene, J. A., Wailoo, K. A., Malina, D., … Marmot, M. G. (2018). Case studies in social medicine: Attending to structural forces in clinical practice. *New England Journal of Medicine*, 379(20), 1958–1961.
Strunin, L., & Boden, L. I. (2004). The workers' compensation system: Worker friend or foe? *American Journal of Industrial Medicine*, 45(4), 338–345.
Stuesse, A. (2016). *Scratching out a living: Latinos, race, and work in the Deep South*. University of California Press.

Stuesse, A. (2018). When they're done with you: Legal violence and structural vulnerability among injured immigrant poultry workers. *Anthropology of Work Review*, 39(2), 79–93.

Stumpf, J. (2006). The crimmigration crisis: Immigrants, crime, and sovereign power. *American University Law Review*, 56(2), 367–419.

Suárez-Orozco, C., & Suárez-Orozco, M. M. (2009). *Children of immigration*. Harvard University Press.

Suårez-Orozco, C., Todorova, I. L., & Louie, J. (2002). Making up for lost time: The experience of separation and reunification among immigrant families. *Family Process*, 41(4), 625–643.

Suárez-Orozco, C., Yoshikawa, H., Teranishi, R., & Suárez-Orozco, M. (2011). Growing up in the shadows: The developmental implications of unauthorized status. *Harvard Educational Review*, 81(3), 438–473.

Subramanian, S. V., Kim, D. J., & Kawachi, I. (2002). Social trust and self-rated health in U.S. communities: A multilevel analysis. *Journal of Urban Health*, 79(1), S21–S34.

Sullivan, M. M., & Rehm, R. (2005). Mental health of undocumented Mexican immigrants: A review of the literature. *Advances in Nursing Science*, 28(3), 240–251.

Sundquist, J., & Johansson, S. E. (1998). The influence of socioeconomic status, ethnicity and lifestyle on body mass index in a longitudinal study. *International Journal of Epidemiology*, 27(1), 57–63.

Sundquist, J., & Winkleby, M. (2000). Country of birth, acculturation status and abdominal obesity in a national sample of Mexican-American women and men. *International Journal of Epidemiology*, 29, 470–477.

Sylla, A., & Cold-Ravnkilde, S. M. (2021). En route to Europe? The anti-politics of deportation from North Africa to Mali. *Geopolitics*, 1–20. DOI: 10.1080/14650045.2021.1995358

Tabak, S., & Levitan, R. (2014). LGBTI migrants in immigration detention: A global perspective. *Harvard Journal of Law and Gender*, 37(1), 513–525.

Tacoli, C. (2009). Crisis or adaptation? Migration and climate change in a context of high mobility. *Environment and urbanization*, 21(2), 1–45.

Talavera, V., Núñez-Mchiri, G. G., & Heyman, J. (2010). Deportation in the U.S.-Mexico borderlands: Anticipation, experience, and memory. In N. De Genova & N. Peutz (Eds.), *The deportation regime* (pp. 166–195). Duke University Press.

Taylor, J. (2003). The story catches you and you fall down: Tragedy, ethnography, and "cultural competence." *Medical Anthropology Quarterly*, 17(2), 159–181.

Thomas, F. (Ed.). (2016). *Handbook of migration and health*. Edward Elgar.

Thornton, C. P., & Veenema, T. G. (2015). Children seeking refuge: A review of the escalating humanitarian crisis of child sexual abuse and HIV/AIDS in Latin America. *Journal of the Association of Nurses in AIDS Care*, 26(4), 432–442.

Thurston, W. E., & Vissandjée, B. (2005). An ecological model for understanding culture as a determinant of women's health. *Critical Public Health*, 15(3), 229–242.

Ticktin, M. I. (2011). *Casualties of care: Immigration and the politics of humanitarianism in France*. University of California Press.

Ticktin, M. (2014). Transnational humanitarianism. *Annual Review of Anthropology*, 43(1), 273–289.

Tober, D. M., Taghdisi, M. H., & Jalali, M. (2006). "Fewer children, better life" or "As many as God wants"? *Medical Anthropology Quarterly*, 20(1), 50–71.

Tormey, A. (2007). "Everyone with eyes can see the problem": Moral citizens and the space of Irish nationhood. *International Migration*, 45(3), 69–100.

Torres, J. M. (2013). Cross-border ties and self-rated health status for young Latino adults in Southern California. *Social Science & Medicine*, 81, 79–86.

Torres, J. M., Deardorff, J., Gunier, R. B., Harley, K. G., Alkon, A., Kogut, K., Eskenazi, B. (2018). Worry about deportation and cardiovascular disease risk factors among adult women: The Center for the Health Assessment of Mothers and Children of Salinas Study. *Annals of Behavioral Medicine*, 52(2), 186–193.

Traylor, A. H., Schmittdiel, J. A., Uratsu, C. S., Mangione, C. M., & U. Subramanian. (2010). Adherence to cardiovascular disease medications: Does patient-provider race/ethnicity and language concordance matter? *Journal of General Internal Medicine*, 25(11), 1172–1177.

UN Economic and Social Council. (2018). Concluding observations on the sixth periodic report of Germany. https://tbinternet.ohchr.org/_layouts/treatybodyexternal/Download.aspx?symbolno=E/C.12/DEU/CO/6&Lang=En

UNHCR. (2021). Refugee data finder. www.unhcr.org/refugee-statistics/

UNICEF. (2016). Nearly 50 million children "uprooted" worldwide. www.unicef.org/press-releases/nearly-50-million-children-uprooted-worldwide

UNICEF. (2017). *A child is a child: Protecting children on the move from violence, abuse and exploitation*. UNICEF.

Valdez, C. R., Padilla, B., & Valentine, J. L. (2013). Consequences of Arizona's immigration policy on social capital among Mexican mothers with unauthorized immigration status. *Hispanic Journal of Behavioral Sciences*, 35(3), 303–322.

Van Herp, M., Parqué, V., Rackley, M., & Ford, N. (2003). Mortality, violence and lack of access to healthcare in the Democratic Republic of Congo. *Disasters*, 27(2), 141–153.

van Osch, E. (2021). "Bad parents", deportable subjects: Borders and deportability in the everyday lives of undocumented families in Belgium. *Journal of Ethnic and Migration Studies*. DOI: https://doi.org/10.1080/1369183X.2021.2015303

Vargas, E. D., & Ybarra, V. D. (2016). U.S. citizen children of undocumented parents: The link between state immigration policy and the health of Latino children. *Journal of Immigrant and Minority Health*, 19(4), 913–920.

Vasey, K., Manderson, L., & Newman, L. (2016). The health and wellbeing of survival migrants. In F. Thomas (Ed.), *Handbook of migration and health*. Edward Elgar.

Vearey, J. (2011). Learning from HIV: Exploring migration and health in South Africa. *Global Public Health*, 7(1), 58–70.

Vearey, J. (2016). Mobility, migration and generalised HIV epidemics: A focus on sub-Saharan Africa. In F. Thomas (Ed.), *Handbook of migration and health* (pp. 340–356). Edward Elgar.

Vearey, J., Modisenyane, M., & Hunter-Adams, J. (2017). Towards a migration-aware health system in South Africa: A strategic opportunity to address health inequity. *South African Health Review*, 2017(1), 89–98.

Viladrich, A. (2012). Beyond welfare reform: Reframing undocumented immigrants' entitlement to health care in the United States, a critical review. *Social Science & Medicine*, 74(6), 822–829.

Viladrich, A. (2018). Botanicas unplugged: Latinos' religious healing and the impact of the immigrant continuum. *African Journal of Traditional, Complementary and Alternative Medicines*, 15(1), 188–198.

Viruell-Fuentes, E. A. (2006). "My heart is always there": The transnational practices of first-generation Mexican immigrant and second-generation Mexican American women. *Identities: Global Studies in Culture and Power*, 13(3), 335–362.

Viruell-Fuentes, E. A., & Schulz, A. J. (2009). Toward a dynamic conceptualization of social ties and context: Implications for understanding immigrant and Latino health. *American Journal of Public Health*, 99(12), 2167–2175.

Vogt, W. (2016). Stuck in the middle with you: The intimate labours of mobility and smuggling along Mexico's migrant route. *Geopolitics*, 21(2), 366–386.

Vogt, W. (2018). *Lives in transit: Violence and intimacy on the migrant journey*. University of California Press.

Walsh, K. (2009). Geographies of the heart in transnational spaces: Love and the intimate lives of British migrants in Dubai. *Mobilities*, 4(3), 427–445.

Walter, N., Bourgois, P., Loinaz, H. M., & Schillinger, D. (2002). Social context of work injury among undocumented day laborers in San Francisco. *Journal of General Internal Medicine*, 17(3), 221–229.

Warner, F. R. (2007). Social support and distress among Q'eqchi' refugee women in Maya Tecún, Mexico. *Medical Anthropology Quarterly*, 21(2), 193–217.

Weiss, R. (2015). *Confronting cultural challenges for migrant healthcare in Switzerland*. Independent Study Project (ISP) Collection. 2104. https://digitalcollections.sit.edu/cgi/viewcontent.cgi?article=3136&context=isp_collection

Wenner, J., Namer, Y., & Razum, O. (2019). Migrants, refugees, asylum seekers: Use and misuse of labels in public health research. In A. Krämer & F. Fischer (Eds.), *Refugee migration and health* (pp. 49–62). Springer.

Wickramage, K., Vearey, J., Zwi, A. B., Robinson, C., & Knipper, M. (2018). Migration and health: A global public health research priority. *BMC Public Health*, 18, 987.

Wild, V., & Dawson, A. (2018). Migration: A core public health ethics issue. *Public Health*, 158, 66–70.

Willen, S. S. (2005). Birthing "Invisible" Children: State power, NGO activism, and reproductive health among "Illegal Migrant" workers in Tel Aviv, Israel. *Journal of Middle East Women's Studies*, 1(2), 55–88.

Willen, S. S. (2007). Toward a critical phenomenology of "illegality": State power, criminalization, and abjectivity among undocumented migrant workers in Tel Aviv, Israel. *International Migration*, 45(3), 8–38.

Willen, S. S. (2010). Citizens, "Real" others, and "Other" others: The biopolitics of otherness and the deportation of unauthorized migrant workers from Tel Aviv, Israel. In N. De Genova & N. Peutz (Eds.), *The deportation regime* (pp. 262–294). Duke University Press.

Willen, S. S. (2012). How is health-related "Deservingness" reckoned? Perspectives from unauthorized im/migrants in Tel Aviv. *Social Science & Medicine*, 74(6), 812–821.

Willen, S. S., Mulligan, J., & Castañeda, H. (2011). Take a stand commentary: How can medical anthropologists contribute to contemporary conversations on "illegal" im/migration and health? *Medical Anthropology Quarterly*, 25(3), 331–356.

Williams, G. A., Odone, A., Tillmann, T., Pharris, A., Oksen, D., Rechel, B., … McKee, M. (2016). Infectious diseases in migrant populations in the European Union and the European Economic Area. In F. Thomas (Ed.), *Handbook of migration and health* (pp. 357–378). Edward Elgar.

Williams, G. H. (2003). The determinants of health: Structure, context and agency. *Sociology of Health and Illness*, 25(3), 131–154.

Wolff, H., Epiney, M., Lourenco, A. P., Costanza, M. C., Delieutraz-Marchand, J., Andreoli, N., … Irion, O. (2008). Undocumented migrants lack access to pregnancy care and prevention. *BMC Public Health*, 8, 93.

Wong, M. (2006). The gendered politics of remittances in Ghanaian transnational families. *Economic Geography*, 82(4), 355–381.

Wong, N. J., Chien, L. C., & Alamgir, H. (2019). Geospatial analysis of refugee access to primary care physicians in San Antonio, Texas. *Journal of Immigrant and Minority Health*, 21(6), 1349–1355.

Woodward, A., Howard, N., & Wolffers, I. (2014). Health and access to care for undocumented migrants living in the European Union: A scoping review. *Health Policy and Planning*, 29(7), 818–830.

World Health Organization. (2007). *International health regulations (2005): Areas of work for implementation.* World Health Organization.

World Health Organization. (2021). www.euro.who.int/en/health-topics/communicable-diseases/tuberculosis/tuberculosis-read-more

Worth, H. (2006). Unconditional hospitality: HIV, ethics and the refugee "problem." *Bioethics*, 20(5), 223–232.

Wright, C. (2003). Moments of emergence: Organizing by and with undocumented and non-citizen people in Canada after September 11. *Refuge*, 3(21), 5–15.

Wurtz, H., & Castañeda, H. (forthcoming). Migration in families and households. In Martina Cvajner, Peter Kivisto & Giuseppe Sciortino (Eds.) *Research handbook on the sociology of migration*. Edward Elgar. Forthcoming.

Xu, Q., & Brabeck, K. (2012). Service utilization for Latino children in mixed-status families. *Social Work Research*, 36(3), 209–221.

Yang, Y. C., Boen, C., Gerken, K., Li, T., Schorpp, K., & Harris, K. M. (2016). Social relationships and physiological determinants of longevity across the human life span. *Proceedings of the National Academy of Sciences*, 113(3), 578–583.

Yarris, K., & Castañeda, H. (2015). Discourses of displacement and deservingness: Interrogating distinctions between economic and forced migration. *International Migration*, 53(3), 64–69.

Yarris, K. E. (2017). *Care across generations: Solidarity and sacrifice in transnational families*. Stanford University Press.

Yea, S. (2017). The art of not being caught: Temporal strategies for disciplining unfree labour in Singapore's contract migration. *Geoforum*, 78, 179–188.

Yoshikawa, H. (2012). *Immigrants raising citizens: Undocumented parents and their young children*. Russell Sage Foundation.

Yoshikawa, H., & Kalil, A. (2011). The effects of parental undocumented status on the developmental contexts of young children in immigrant families. *Child Development Perspectives*, 5(4), 291–297.

Zayas, L. H. (2010). Protecting citizen-children safeguards our common future. *Journal of Health Care for the Poor and Underserved*, 21(3), 809–814.

Zunzunegui, M.V., Koné, A., Johri, M., Béland, F., Wolfson, C., & Bergman, H. (2004). Social networks and self-rated health in two French-speaking Canadian community dwelling populations over 65. *Social Science and Medicine*, 58(10), 2069–2081.

INDEX

access to healthcare: alternative strategies 56; barriers other than policies 52–53; bureaucratic disentitlement 55; critical perspectives 48–49; deportation fears and 108; deservingness 48; exclusions 48; families, impact of lack of access on 53–54; gatekeeping 54–55; humanitarian models 51; international conventions and 48; legal status and 46–47; low rates of 130; policy frameworks and 49–52; refugees and asylum seekers 121–123; spillover effects due to lack of 53–54; United States 49–51; universal health care systems 51–52; variations within countries 52; via charities and NGOs 55–56
acculturation, health of migrants and 26–29
adverse childhood events 110
Alabama Taxpayer and Citizen Protection Act 50
ambiguous loss 110
Arizona Senate Bill 1070 50
arrival, health and 6
assimilation, health of migrants and 26–29
asylum seekers: access to healthcare 121–123; barriers to care after 117; camps 120; children 119; crisis in Hessen, Germany 116–117; critical perspectives 118–119; definitions 118; deservingness and 123; different health beliefs 123–124; financial stress 122; food insecurity 124; gender 119; health issues 117, 123–124; levels of 2; medical examinations 121; mental health 124–125; proof of torture and persecution 121; protracted displacement 119–121; racialization 123; resettlement and integration services 122; resilience and 119; structural invisibility 118; trauma history checklists 121; unique health needs 123–124
attachment theory 110
Australia: externalization of border controls 41; reception centers 120–121

backstretch workers 80–81
behavioural explanations, move to structural approaches 29–31
Belgium, access to and utilization of healthcare in 51
bi/multinational approaches 7
biomedical perspective 64
borders: abolition of 130; communicable disease 71, 78; COVID-19 pandemic 75–77; critical border studies 12–14; externalization of border controls 40–41; internalized controls 39, 41; as phenomenological events 14; problematizing 13–14; as processes 13; as reified object 13; respatialization of 39–42; rethinking 14; sovereign territory and 13; unequal experiences of 13; violence of 35–36
bureaucratic disentitlement 55

camps 120
caregiving, transnational 44

charities: access to healthcare via 55–56; referral networks 58
children: cross-border ties 44–45; deportation 110–112; detention process 110; familial shifts and separations 42–43; future research 132; parental deportation 114; refugees and asylum seekers 119; undocumented 99; violence at borders 36
chronicities 85
citizenship: critical perspectives 15, 17; reproduction and 97–98
civic life, lack of 106
climate change 133
clinical encounters: barriers in 60; biomedical perspective 64; communication barriers 61–62; critical perspectives 60–61; cultural competency 62–64; cultural humility 64; cultural mediation 65–66; culture concept, use of 63–64; diversity in the clinical workforce 66; diversity sensitivity 62–64; exclusion 58–59; explanatory models of illness 62–63; Gheorghe example 58–59, 60; health literacy 65–66; interpreters, use of in 61–62; language barriers 61–62; migration aware whole system approaches 66; pain assessment 90; patient-centeredness 62–64; social context 60–61; structural competency 64–65; workers' compensation and 89–90
colonial legacies 70–71
communicable disease: borders 71, 78; colonial legacies 70–71; COVID-19 75–79; critical perspectives 70; HIV/AIDS 73–75; Morocco, sub-Saharan Africans in 68–69; movements of populations, information on 69–70; risk for migrants 70; stigmatization of communities 71–72; tuberculosis 72–73
communication barriers in clinical encounters 61–62
communities: deportation, impact of 113; lack of access to healthcare 54
community health workers 65–66
Costa Rica, access to and utilization of healthcare in 52
COVID-19 pandemic: as disrupter of migration 2–3; internal mobility controls 76–77; longer-term impact 78; migrants in host countries 77–78; mobility, management of human 75–79; Morocco, sub-Saharan Africans in 68–69; research agenda after 133–134; as security threat 77; stigmatization of communities 72; transit sites, migrants in 78
criminal law, immigration law and 105
criminals, migrants seen as 36
crisis, migration referred to as 19
critical border studies 12–14
critical perspectives: access to and utilization of healthcare 48–49; borders 12–14; broadening of lens through 3; citizenship 15, 17; clinical encounters 60–61; communicable disease 70; contexts 3; critical border studies 12–14; defined 3; deportation 105–107; deportation regimes 16; detention 105–107; enforcement 105–107; forced displacement 118–119; gender 95; on health 21–25; illegality 15–16; inequality 4; labor 82–85; marginalization 4; migrant health 3–5; moving forward 127–129; occupational health 82–85; origins and reasons for migration 4; precarity 16; problematization of understandings 4; refugees and asylum seekers 118–119; rethinking understandings 3; sexuality 95; social context 60–61; structural approaches, move from behavioural explanations to 29–31; transit, health in 34–35
critical public health approaches 21–22
cross-border ties 43–45
cultural competency of clinicians 62–64
cultural humility 64
cultural mediation 65–66
culture concept, use of 63–64
cumulative risk perspective 111

decompensation, workers' 87–89
defining global issue, migration as 2–3
Denmark 56
dental issues 59
deportation: access to healthcare and 108; children 110–112; communities, impact on 113; critical perspectives 16, 105–107; families, impact on 112–113; fear of 107; feeling of deportability 106; health issues during 109–110; impact on well-being 104; masculinity and 99–100; outsourcing of 105; parental 114; physical health, deportability and 108; pyramid 106–107; return to country of origin 113–114; self-deportation 106
deservingness: access to healthcare 48; compensation for workplace injuries and 89; concept of 24–25; ethnic

discrimination 59; inclusion/exclusion and 30; legal violence 54; refugees and asylum seekers 123
detention: critical perspectives 105–107; health issues during 109–110; impact on well-being 104; prolonged 119–121
developed countries, focus on migration to 8
developing countries, refugees in 120–121
diabetes 23, 30–31
disabilities from workplace injuries 90–91
disease *see* communicable disease
diversity in the clinical workforce 66
diversity sensitivity 62–64

education, medical 65
enforcement: critical perspectives 105–107; familial vulnerability 106; impact on well-being 104; internal practices 103–104; local levels 105–106; pathogenic law enforcement 106; raids on homes and workplaces 109; *see also* deportation
ethnic discrimination: deservingness and 59; pain assessment 90
ethnic resemblance in the clinical workforce 66
European Union (EU): externalization of border controls 40–41; militarization of border 35–36
exceptionalization of migration, refraining from 129–130
explanatory models of illness 62–63
externalization of border controls 40–41, 105

faciality 83–84
familial shifts and separations 95–96; cross-border ties 43–45; deportation 110–112; during transit 42–43
familial vulnerability 106
families: deportation, impact of 112–113; lack of access to healthcare 53–54
family planning, migration and 96
fathers 99–100
feminist approach 95
fertility patterns 97
food insecurity 124
forced displacement: access to healthcare 121–123; barriers to care after 117; children and youth 119; critical perspectives 118–119; definitions 118; in developing countries 120–121; financial stress 122; health issues 117, 123–124; levels of 2; medical examinations 121; mental health 124–125; proof of torture and persecution 121; protracted displacement 119–121; reception centers 120–121; resettlement and integration services 122; resilience and 119; structural invisibility 118; trauma history checklists 121; unique health needs 123–124
forced immobility 37–38
fragmented journeys 37–38
France, access to and utilization of healthcare in 52
freedom of movement 14–15, 17, 130
FRONTEX 40
future research 130–134

gatekeeping, access to healthcare and 54–55
gender: critical perspectives 95, 96; cross-border ties 44–45; familial shifts and separations 95–96; family planning, migration and 96; fathers 99–100; fertility patterns 97; geographies of power 95; HIV/AIDS 74–75; labor and occupational health 84; marriage, migration and 96; masculinities 99–100; paternity 98; pregnancy, migrant health and 92–94, 97; refugees and asylum seekers 119; reproduction and 97–98; violence at borders 36
geographies of power, gendered 95
Germany: access to and utilization of healthcare 51, 56; Maternity Protection Act 1968 93–94; pregnancy, migrant health and 93–94; racialization of migrants 20
global issue, migration as 2–3
global policies 129

hazards in the workplace 85–86
health. critical perspectives on 21–25
health literacy 65–66
healthy migrant effect 25–26
HIV/AIDS: management 75; Southern Africa 73–74; stigmatization of communities 71–72, 73; structural causes 74–75; vulnerability to, migration and 73–74
home communities: health profile of 5–6; return to 6
home raids 109
humanitarianism, deservingness and 24–25
human rights, deservingness and 24–25

Illegal Immigration Reform and Immigrant Responsibility Act (US) 49–50

illegality: access to and utilization of healthcare 48; criminals, migrants seen as 36; critical perspectives 15–16; labor and occupational health 84–85
il/legal status, historical processes and 18
illiegalization, processes of 18
immigrant health paradox 26
immigrants, 'migrants' as preferred term 17–18
immigration as social determinant of health 22
immobility: forced 37–38; future research 132
incorporation into host society, health of migrants and 26–29
India, shoot-to-kill practices at borders 36
inequality: critical perspectives 4; pathogenic role of social 30; social 21–22; structural approaches, move from behavioural explanations to 29–30
infectious diseases *see* communicable disease
infrastructural determinants of health 24
injuries at the workplace 87–91
internalization of border controls 39, 41, 105
internal migration 8
interpreters, use of in clinical encounters 61–62
intersectionality: acculturation, health of migrants and 27; migrants 18
intimate partner violence 101–102
involuntary/voluntary migrants 2
Italy, access to and utilization of healthcare in 51

kafala system 84–85

labor: abuses 86–87; chronicities 85; compensation systems 87–89; critical perspectives 82–85; decompensation, workers' 87–89; deservingness, compensation and 89; disabilities from workplace injuries 90–91; faciality 83–84; gender and 84; hazards in the workplace 85–86; illegality, condition of 84–85; injuries 87–91; international conventions 82; kafala system 84–85; legal violence 84; legitimacy of compensation claims 89; life course perspective 85; mutual aid societies 87; negative tropes about migrants 83–84; obstruction of compensation claims 88; pain assessment 90; racetrack work in the US 80–81; search for work 81; segregation by ethnicity and legality 84; structural approaches 82–85; structural vulnerability 83, 84; syndemics 85; temporality 88; trafficking 86; wage theft 86–87
language barriers in clinical encounters 61–62
law, immigration 15
legal status: access to healthcare and 46–47; sexual health 101
legal violence 54, 84; family separation through deportation 112
legitimacy of workplace injuries 89
LGBTQ+ migrations 100; detention process 110
life course perspective 85
liminal legality 16
literacy, health 65–66
local policies 131

marginalization, critical perspectives on 4
marriage, migration and 96
masculinities 99–100
Maternity Protection Act 1968, Germany 93–94
mediation, cultural 65–66
mental health of refugees and asylum seekers 124–125
methodology: bi-/multinational approaches 7; challenges of 6–7; nationalism, methodological 6; varied, across disciplines 7
Mexico to US migration 32–33, 35, 40
migrants: definitions 18; intersectionality 18; as preferred term 17–18
migration aware whole system approaches 66
militarization of borders 35–36
mixed status families 99; gender roles and 95–96
Morocco: COVID-19 pandemic 68, 69; progressive reforms re. migrants 69; sub-Saharan Africans in 68–69
movement phase of migration *see* transit phase of migration
multi/binational approaches 7
mutual aid societies 87

nationalism, methodological 6
nationhood, reproduction and 97–98
navigators, health care 65–66
necroviolence 36
Netherlands, access to and utilization of healthcare in 51

non-governmental organizations (NGOs): access to healthcare via 55–56; referral networks 58
Northern countries as preferred destinations 17
number of migrants 2

obesity, migration and 28–29
occupational health: abuses 86–87; chronicities 85; critical perspectives 82–85; decompensation, workers' 87–89; deservingness, compensation and 89; disabilities from workplace injuries 90–91; faciality 83–84; gender and 84; hazards in the workplace 85–86; illegality, condition of 84–85; injuries 87–91; international conventions 82; kafala system 84–85; legal violence 84; legitimacy of compensation claims 89; life course perspective 85; mutual aid societies 87; negative tropes about migrants 83–84; obstruction of compensation claims 88; pain assessment 90; racetrack work in the US 80–81; segregation by ethnicity and legality 84; structural approaches 82–85; structural vulnerability 83, 84; syndemics 85; temporality 88; trafficking 86; wage theft 86–87
oral health 59
origins and reasons for migration 4
'others,' disease and 70–71
outsourcing: of border controls 40–41; deportation 105

pain assessment 90
pandemics *see* communicable disease; COVID-19 pandemic
parenthood: consequences of 97; transnational families 99–100
paternity 98
pathogenic law enforcement 106
Personal Responsibility and Work Opportunity Reconciliation Act (PRWORA) 49–50
policies: global 129; local 131
positionality, researcher 17
post-traumatic stress disorder (PTSD) 124–125
power, gendered geographies of 95
precarity 16
preferences, system of 15
pregnancy, migrant health and 92–94, 97
problematization of understandings 4
process of migration, moments of 5–6
protracted displacement 119–121
pyramid, deportation 106–107

queer migrations 100; detention process 110

racetrack work in the US 80–81
racialization of migrants 19–20; criminals, migrants seen as 36; hierarchies of 59; refugees and asylum seekers 123; reproduction and 97
racism, socioeconomic status and 30
raids on homes and workplaces 109
reasons for migration 4
reception centers 120–121
refugees: access to healthcare 121–123; barriers to care after 117; camps 120; children 119; critical perspectives 118–119; definitions 19, 118; deservingness and 123; in developing countries 120–121; different health beliefs 123–124; financial stress 122; food insecurity 124; gender 119; health issues 117, 123–124; levels of 2; medical examinations 121; mental health 124–125; proof of torture and persecution 121; protracted displacement 119–121; racialization 123; reception centers 120–121; resettlement and integration services 122; resilience and 119; structural invisibility 118; trauma history checklists 121; unique health needs 123–124
remittances 43, 44–45
reproduction: gender and 97–98; transnational parenting 98–99; undocumented children 99
reproduction, migrant health and 92–94
research, future 130–134
researcher positionality 17
resilience: future research 132; refugees and asylum seekers 119
respatialization of border controls 39–42
return to home communities 6, 113–114; medical 20–21

San Francisco 52
SARS epidemic 72
securitization practices 39–40, 105
self-deportation 106
settings for healthcare *see* clinical encounters
sex trafficking, overemphasis on 38

sexual health 100–101
sexuality: critical perspectives 95, 96; family planning, migration and 96; fathers 99–100; fertility patterns 97; marriage, migration and 96; masculinities 99–100; paternity 98; pregnancy, migrant health and 92–94, 97; queer migrations 100; reproduction 97–98
smuggling and trafficking 38–39
social capital 28
social context, clinical encounters and 60–61
social determinants of health 22
social inequalities 21–22
social medicine 21
social sciences 22
Southern Africa, HIV/AIDS and 73–74
South-South migration 8
sovereign territory, borders and 13
Spain: access to and utilization of healthcare 51, 55; access to healthcare 52
stigmatization of communities 71–72
stratified reproduction 97
street-level bureaucrats 55
structural approaches: HIV/AIDS 74–75; labor and occupational health 82–85; move from behavioural explanations to 29–31
structural competency 64–65
structural invisibility 118
structural violence 23, 101
structural vulnerability 23, 83, 84
stuckness 37–38
Switzerland, access to healthcare in 52
syndemics 23, 85
system of preferences 15

temporary legality 16
terminology, importance of 17–18
toxic stress 110
trafficking 38–39, 86
transit phase of migration: borders, violence of 35–36; broader context for 34; COVID-19 pandemic 78; critical approaches 34–35; critical perspectives 34–35; cross-border ties 43–45; familial shifts and separations 42–43; forced immobility 37–38; health during 6; Mexico to US migration 32–33; respatialization of border controls 39–42; sending/host countries, blurring of 35; smuggling and trafficking 38–39; transit countries 37–38
transnational families: fathers 99–100; gender roles and 95–96; parenting and 99–100
travel *see* transit phase of migration
tuberculosis 72–73

United States: access to and utilization of healthcare 49–51, 52; access to healthcare, legal status and 46–47; Alabama Taxpayer and Citizen Protection Act 50; Arizona Senate Bill 1070 50; enforcement, internal practices of 103–104; externalization of border controls 40; Illegal Immigration Reform and Immigrant Responsibility Act 49–50; internalization of border controls 41; Mexico to US migration 32–33, 35, 40; Personal Responsibility and Work Opportunity Reconciliation Act (PRWORA) 49–50; policy frameworks for healthcare 49–51; Proposition 187; California 49, 50; racetrack work in 80–81; racialization of migrants 20; resettlement and integration services 122; San Francisco 52; spillover effects due to lack of access to healthcare 53–54; violence of borders 35
utilization of healthcare: alternative strategies 56; barriers other than policies 52–53; bureaucratic disentitlement 55; critical perspectives 48–49; deportation fears and 108; deservingness 48; exclusions 48; families, impact of lack of access on 53–54; gatekeeping 54–55; humanitarian models 51; illegality and 48; international conventions and 48; legal status and 46–47; policy frameworks and 49–52; spillover effects due to lack of 53–54; United States 49–51; universal health care systems 51–52; variations within countries 52; via charities and NGOs 55–56

violence: of borders 35–36; intimate partner violence 101–102; legal 54, 84, 112; necroviolence 36; structural 23, 101
visa access 14–15
voluntary/involuntary migrants 2
vulnerability: familial 106; HIV/AIDS 73–74; structural 23, 83, 84

wage theft 86–87
work *see* labor

For Product Safety Concerns and Information please contact our EU representative GPSR@taylorandfrancis.com
Taylor & Francis Verlag GmbH, Kaufingerstraße 24, 80331 München, Germany

www.ingramcontent.com/pod-product-compliance
Ingram Content Group UK Ltd.
Pitfield, Milton Keynes, MK11 3LW, UK
UKHW020138200926
475702UK00005B/802
* 9 7 8 1 1 3 8 4 9 0 4 2 0 *